W9-AIV-364

"Alec is dedicated and passionate about seeking greatness in all he does, and about helping others reach their full potential through hard work and an open heart."

—Derek Hough, *New York Times* bestselling author and Emmy Award–winning performer

"We have no doubt *Seven Sundays* will transform your temple and your walk with the Lord. Alec will encourage you, he will challenge you, and most of all, he will teach you how God can transform and renew your temple and soul."

—Carlos and Alexa PenaVega

"After meeting and working with Alec, I can see the passion and love that he embodies. He is a truly inspirational young man whose spirit will inspire everyone he touches. I have no doubt that this book will affect many lives!"

—Cheryl Ladd, actress, author, and entrepreneur

SEVEN SUNDAYS

A FAITH, FITNESS, AND FOOD PLAN FOR
LASTING SPIRITUAL AND PHYSICAL CHANGE

Alec Penix
and MYATT MURPHY

HOWARD BOOKS

New York   London   Toronto   Sydney   New Delhi

HOWARD
B O O K S

An Imprint of Simon & Schuster, Inc.
1230 Avenue of the Americas
New York, NY 10020

Copyright © 2018 by Alec Penix and Myatt Murphy

This publication contains the opinions and ideas of its author. It is intended to provide helpful and informative material on the subjects addressed in the publication. It is sold with the understanding that the author and publisher are not engaged in rendering medical, health, or any other kind of personal professional services in the book. The reader should consult his or her medical, health, or other competent professional before adopting any of the suggestions in this book or drawing inferences from it.

The author and publisher specifically disclaim all responsibility for any liability, loss, or risk, personal or otherwise, that is incurred as a consequence, directly or indirectly, of the use and application of any of the contents of this book.

First Howard Books hardcover edition December 2018

HOWARD and colophon are trademarks of Simon & Schuster, Inc.

For information about special discounts for bulk purchases, please contact Simon & Schuster Special Sales at 1-866-506-1949 or business@simonandschuster.com.

The Simon & Schuster Speakers Bureau can bring authors to your live event. For more information or to book an event, contact the Simon & Schuster Speakers Bureau at 1-866-248-3049 or visit our website at www.simonspeakers.com.

Interior design by Bryden Spevak

Manufactured in the United States of America

10 9 8 7 6 5 4 3 2

Library of Congress Cataloging-in-Publication Data has been applied for.

ISBN 978-1-5011-8985-2
ISBN 978-1-5011-8986-9 (ebook)

I want to dedicate this book to those who have gathered the courage within themselves to take a leap of faith toward bettering their lives. I know change can seem daunting at times, but I truly believe that with faith, anything is possible. I look forward to going on this journey with each and every one of you.

CONTENTS

SEVEN SUNDAYS

FROM FIT TO FOUND

Without His love, I was half a man, even though to others, I seemed complete.

As a premier celebrity trainer in Los Angeles, I've spent the last decade working with actors, models, professional athletes, Olympians, dancers, film and television executives, CEOs, and musicians. But as successful as I've become in the field of fitness, moving to Tinseltown initially began as a journey to prove something—to others, but especially to myself.

My childhood wasn't the best environment for building self-esteem. I was abandoned by my mother at the age of five, and I also suffered from a learning disability throughout my school years. Because my disability made me different, all I wanted to do was fit in with my peers. So I found something I was good at—sports—and decided to work out harder than everyone to paint an image of myself as a jock. It was an image that would become the foundation of my life until God would eventually break me free from it.

The lack of love and security in my life left me constantly depressed and obsessed with the physical, the only thing I felt I had any control over. Growing up, I sought out external things to make myself feel happy and fulfilled and spent my entire life staying in top shape. My search for happiness even helped shape the career I would eventually pursue. While I was receiving my degree in dietetics at the University of Kentucky, I dreamed of becoming a celebrity trainer in Hollywood, and I eventually made my way to Los Angeles to work with top celebrities. But I had chased happiness all the way to Hollywood only to have it continue to elude me, no matter how hard I tried to catch it.

What I didn't know at the time was that the real reason I felt called to LA was that God was orchestrating my steps to salvation.

It wasn't easy initially. Working as a trainer at a corporate gym, sleeping on the floor in a one-bedroom apartment, and living with three guys wasn't ideal for me, but I knew I had to stick with it. I eventually broke off from the gym to start my own business. At the time, I only had a few clients, but eventually my big break happened—I was going on tour as the trainer for the band Big Time Rush.

From that point, the momentum started, and I thought I would finally find that love and security I was hoping to have in my life. After all, I wasn't just a busy trainer—I was now a "celebrity" trainer. And very quickly, I found myself working with gold medalists, professional dancers, artists, musicians—you name it. Yet despite having what most may define as examples of success (being physically fit and having a thriving business working with celebrities), my lack of self-worth continued to prevent me from appreciating what I had achieved. I continued to struggle with depression for several years until I started to notice something—or should I say Him.

When I first found Christ, He was working through specific clients I was training. One by one, I began to notice that the people who were succeeding physically were also deeply connected to their faith. Each was indirectly showing me what I was personally missing out on and how my soul was malnourished. Each had this overwhelming sense of unselfishness about them—what I would call the "essence of God"—and that unselfishness convicted me of my own selfishness.

Those of the faith seemed to have so much to give of themselves, and yet, there I was, struggling just to get through the day. Each one gave more to me in every session than I could give to them—and I was their trainer. I couldn't help but wonder why my tank was always on empty.

The lack of God in my life became ever more evident as my depression continued to worsen. Until one day, alone in a hotel room, at a point where I had finally hit rock bottom with my lifelong battle with despair . . .

. . . God took custody of me.

I found myself in bed, unsure of how I even got there, hungover and trying to remember what had happened the night before. All I could put together were flashes and fragments, each remembered moment leaving me so incredibly embarrassed that I didn't leave my room all day.

My friends were calling me—some even came and knocked on my door—but I was so ashamed of myself, I didn't want to be seen. I made the right decision, because on that day, I had encountered God.

I tell everyone that God apprehended me, although I do understand that God forcing us to know Him isn't really how it works. But I felt as if a voice was saying to me: It is time to become the man that I've called you to be. It was Jesus—He was what I was missing all along. And at that very moment, just as we are told in Hebrews 3:15—that if you hear His voice, do not harden your heart—I chose to listen. And I told Him yes, I'm all-in.

And since that day, all-in is where I have remained—and I've been running toward my destiny ever since. I knew my path was going to be different. From that moment, I was on fire for the Lord, and I knew in my heart from the very beginning that I was put on this earth to share something special with the world.

With His love, all the pieces started to come together, and I started to understand why I had always failed to appreciate what I had accomplished and why I was blindly seeking perfection within myself. I finally began to understand that I had the power to release and heal what had always held me back, and that I was ready to embrace what would move me forward. I was finally on this journey toward becoming whole—to becoming happy—and that led to me completely changing how I trained both myself and my clients.

Before receiving God's grace, I came at health and fitness from a very shallow perspective. I was chasing the money, fame, and reputation I thought would come, not knowing at the time that my motives were shallow. There wasn't much attempt to build any type of relationship, and I never thought of helping my clients spiritually or emotionally, because at the time, I couldn't even help myself. It was always about getting clients in shape and then getting them on their way.

But after embracing Jesus, I began to speak, act, and think differently. One of the most memorable moments during my transition came at a totally unexpected time. I was asked to speak about my testimony at a small group that was hosted by my peers. They were so moved by my passion and newfound love for life that they asked me to come back to speak. I found myself beginning to share that same testimony with just about anyone, especially my clients. I started saying things that some Christians would be hesitant to say, but I wasn't just any Christian—through Him, I was fearless. I started to sound like the believer I had become and would say things like: "I surrender to God," "God has given me life," and "I'm on fire for the Lord." I wasn't ashamed, because I knew in my heart it was real—and it continues to be today.

That enthusiasm found its way into my work with clients, and I began focusing more on their hearts and minds; my experience and knowledge about exercise and nutrition were just the cherry on top. I wanted our connection to be more relational than transactional. I cared about them as people rather than as clients. Most important, I cared about *all* of them rather than just a part of them—and began to approach fitness from a "faith first" perspective.

Because of the encounter I had with Jesus, my vision suddenly became clear, and I knew what God was doing in me and through me—and that began to affect people. I became more passionate and less indifferent. I felt like a victor and not a victim, and started to live in love and not fear. With clients, I now had a relationship in which I wasn't merely their trainer but became their friend and their rock—someone to turn to for advice, love, and support. I stopped being timid and grew bolder, asking them questions whenever I saw something in their lives that was burdening them and taking its toll both physically and spiritually.

The questions were never things I thought out beforehand; they were questions that came to mind inspired by the Holy Spirit. But no matter what I found myself asking, I was always trying to get my clients to look inward, to inspire them to look at their situation from a different perspective. I asked questions like:

- Why do you feel that way?
- Why do you think this is a habit for you?
- What is holding you back?
- Why are you being so hard on yourself?
- How can I help you in this area?
- What do you need from me?

My approach evolved into one in which I sought to help people not only look their best but also feel—and be—their best. I started focusing on a client's "interior" first by addressing their individual spiritual needs, knowing how that would aid their "physical" transformation by breaking down whatever internal roadblocks were in their way. At the same time, I began to feed their spirit through words, actions, and activities that helped change the way they looked at fitness so that it became more than merely a means to an end. With some clients, it was finding simple words of encouragement to get them through their day. With others, I felt it was appropriate to bring up scriptures or stories in the Bible that were applicable to their situations. But the most important lesson that I learned—the action I felt most drawn toward doing—was the art of listening.

And then something incredible happened.

Not only were my clients getting in shape faster, but they found it much easier to stick with my program when I wasn't with them. Living a healthier lifestyle was no longer about *having* to lose fifteen pounds for a tour, musical, or movie role. Instead it became about *wanting* to lose fifteen pounds because of the positive impact the journey (not necessarily the end result) would have on their life and those around them.

I finally understood that living a healthy lifestyle is much easier when we also build a deeper relationship with Jesus. That by combining faith and fitness, my clients had an easier time trying to reach the physical goals they had for themselves, and they also started to feel more fulfilled and see spiritual growth as well. For it's through His love that we find a different source of strength, one that allows us to not only make it through and succeed but unlock an inner beauty that comes out on the outside as well.

I had always felt there was something more living within me, something that wanted to come out and be expressed—but I just didn't know how to do that. I finally realized the reason it was so difficult for me to share it with the world was fear. But as I began to start seeing myself through God's eyes, I was able to build a newfound love for myself and finally understood that I was worthy of expressing this part of me. I finally found not what I *thought* I needed, but what I *truly* needed—the love and security He offers each and every one of us.

The Seven Sundays program is a culmination of what worked for me and what works for my clients. It's also the beginning of your journey, one that will bring you closer to Him and, through that bond, even closer to a healthier, happy life.

After Seven Sundays, you will be fitter and stronger than when you started. But it's not just your body that will dramatically change as a result. So many other aspects of your life will change as well. You'll begin to eat and sleep better, and your life will be richer in both positive experiences and healthier relationships. You'll discover a confidence within yourself as you step outside your comfort zone to achieve things that once seemed impossible. You'll learn to love and appreciate what's around you more than ever before, and perhaps discover blessings you never noticed that have always been all around you. You'll make a profound difference in your church and in the lives of so many people, from those closest to you to some you may never have the pleasure to meet. But, most important, you'll connect with God on a level you may never have thought imaginable.

PART ONE

Why All Things *Are* Possible

I

WHY IS CARING FOR YOURSELF SO HARD?

*Beloved, I pray that in every way you may succeed and prosper
and be in good health, just as your soul prospers.*
—3 JOHN 1:2

Have you ever wondered why it's so hard to make changes to your lifestyle, even though you know how much richer your life would be if you did?

Have you ever noticed how so many people see healthy living as something they *have* to do, not something they want to do?

Have you ever been confused when someone who looks great still seems so dissatisfied with their "perfect" body—and so unhappy with themselves?

Have you ever tried to lose weight, to build your physical strength, or to get healthier, but gotten discouraged and given up?

Why is it so hard to care for yourself, even if you really want to?

Throughout my own life, as well as my career as a celebrity trainer,

I've found that there are all kinds of reasons Christians struggle to lead a healthy lifestyle. Sometimes the reason is practical—they lack something they need, whether it's time, money, space, or something else, and that makes it hard to keep up with their fitness program. But I have found that often the reasons people struggle to stick with a program for healthy living are deeper than that. Sometimes people are driven by feelings of unworthiness, while others spend so much time caring for others that they don't have the time or energy—or even the permission—to care for themselves. Have you ever said or thought something along these lines?

I DON'T HAVE ENOUGH TIME

We all have too many demands on our time. You may be working multiple jobs, be caring for children or parents, or spending every spare moment volunteering at your church or in other ways. You are no doubt doing everything you can just to keep your head above water. I get that. But in the end, we all make time for the things that are important to us. We generally find a way to make time for the things we love to do, and it's hard to prioritize the things that feel like chores. The good news is that living a healthier lifestyle doesn't actually require any more time than any of us have. In fact, experts agree that it takes only a minimum of 150 minutes of aerobic exercise a week to reap results. That's just two and a half hours a week! Throughout this book, we'll be looking at ways to turn what you may think of as a chore—exercising, getting enough sleep, cooking healthy meals—into activities you genuinely enjoy. If you can you do that, you'll always find the time to prioritize the things that will make you healthier.

I'M TOO OLD TO START EXERCISING

Maybe you've never worked out a day in your life. That's okay! The truth is, the older you are, the *more* benefit you'll get from working out. Exercise prevents bone loss,[1] improves balance and coordination, boosts both memory[2] and mood, makes you stronger, and lowers your risk of various chronic conditions and health problems, such as hypertension,[3] arthritis,[4] diabetes,[5] and even cancer.[6]

FOCUSING ON MYSELF MAKES ME FEEL VAIN

I've noticed that Christians sometimes have a hard time letting themselves focus on their own needs. We often have a sense that we're supposed to be using our time to serve others. But when we don't take care of ourselves, we're never able to bring as much energy and effort to those we care for. Also, when all we do is give, give, give, it can put us in starvation mode. We eventually reach a point where we have nothing left to give.

I'M NOT STRONG ENOUGH TO STICK IT OUT

How many times have you traveled the path toward a healthy lifestyle, only to find yourself stopping halfway? Maybe it's happened enough times that you wonder if there's any point in trying again.

When clients come to me with that outlook, I ask them why they don't believe in themselves. We dig into it, and we try to uncover the fear that is triggering that doubt in them. And in all honesty, it almost always comes down to one thing—they're afraid to fail. They don't give it their all because they don't want to let themselves—or someone else—down. Who are you afraid to let down? Why are you afraid to give it a shot? My clients usually come to understand that you have to be able to risk failure if you want to have any chance of succeeding.

EXERCISE IS BORING, AND HEALTHY FOOD IS BLAND

While it's true that some of the changes you'll need to make to eat better, become fitter, and live a healthy life can take some adjusting to, that doesn't mean they have to be boring. To keep things interesting, you have to mix things up and try new things every single day. There are so many activities, flavors, and experiences in the world that fit into a healthy lifestyle; it's simply a matter of knowing how to keep things interesting for both your body and your soul.

I DON'T DESERVE IT

When we feel unworthy of accepting something positive, such as happiness or health, it's because we don't love ourselves. We end up accepting only what we think we deserve.

Recognizing that you warrant the effort it takes to get healthy is something that has to come from within. You have to believe wholeheartedly that you are worth it so you can acknowledge and receive what you rightfully deserve.

In times like this, we can always turn to Jesus as a reminder of who we are and who we belong to. Two of my favorite scriptures to read whenever I feel like this include:

And if children, heirs also: heirs of God and fellow heirs with Christ, if indeed we share in His suffering so that we may also share in His glory.

—ROMANS 8:17

And now I commend you to God and to the word of His grace. His grace is able to build you up and to give you the inheritance among all those who are sanctified.

—ACTS 20:32

You may not love yourself—not yet, at least—but you can trust God, and your history does not have to define your destiny. Remind yourself that we have inherited royalty for what Christ sacrificed on the cross.

I HATE MY BODY

There are many people out there who others would say are incredibly fit and healthy, but they still don't love themselves the way they should. They never let themselves see what's apparent to everyone around them. They never believe that their body—sculpted and polished as it may be—is good enough. The only way these people will ever see that they are good enough is if they take the focus off the physical and start to work on other parts of themselves. You can lose all the weight you want to, have a perfect diet, and feel fantastic—but that's still not a guarantee you'll love your body. To get there, you have to move beyond the physical.

I was once part of that congregation of people who couldn't appreciate what they had. I struggled for years to believe that my body was good enough, strong enough, lean enough. I know firsthand—through both personal experience and working with my clientele—what it's like to see your body through the wrong lens.

Whatever shape you are in, your body is the temple of God, and that alone means it's good enough. Through the course of this book, we're going to spend as much time building up your spirit as we do building up your body. Through a deeper relationship with Him, I hope you'll come to see that your physical body is worthy of love and respect, and that through God all things are possible.

EATING HEALTHY IS TOO EXPENSIVE

Many people believe that good-for-you foods are pricier than fare that may not be as healthy, but have you ever put it to the test? I'm willing to bet that certain unhealthy foods—such as high-priced lattes and energy bars—may cost more than healthy foods and drinks you could be substituting for them.

However, I will confess that a landmark study showed that the cost of eating an extremely healthy diet—full of fish, fruits, nuts, and vegetables—is roughly $1.50 per day higher than eating an unhealthy diet of processed foods and refined grains.[7] That does add up over time.

How much is your health worth? Eating healthier can minimize your risk of so many chronic diseases, make you feel more energized, and boost your immune system so that you're less likely to be sick. Is one-quarter of what you probably spend on a cup of coffee worth it? I know that it is.

And how much are you wasting when it comes to what you eat? According to the US Department of Agriculture, the average family of four wastes nearly $1,500 worth of food each year.[8] That said, all it may take—if cost is that much of a consideration—is just being a little wiser in how often you purchase perishable foods so that you're less likely to throw away food that may have spoiled or gone past its expiration date.

2

YOU MUST SURRENDER TO SUCCEED

So many diet, weight loss, and lifestyle programs concentrate on nurturing and strengthening the *physical* body. But what most, if not all, tend to neglect is the importance of nurturing and enhancing the *spiritual* body, equally and simultaneously.

When we focus purely on the physical, we either fumble through or fail, or feel unsatisfied, even when we succeed. That's because no matter how fit we may wish to be or eventually become, if we ignore our spirit in the process, it's impossible to ever feel truly fulfilled.

I truly witnessed God's work in my life in this area. I worked extremely hard on my body for many years, always thinking that the better I looked, the better my life would be. The contradictory thing was that the harder I worked, the unhappier I became. But God showed me that I was much more than a physical being, and that's when everything began to change. Once I started to put more emphasis on strengthening my spirit, slowly but surely, wholeness was in my sights.

Our physical body is nothing more than a vessel. It's a vessel we may be able to shape and build, but it's a vessel nonetheless. It's just there to carry something inside, as 1 Corinthians 6:19 reminds us:

Do you not know that your body is a temple of the Holy Spirit who is within you, whom you have from God, and that you are not your own?

For most of my life, I had molded my vessel through diet and exercise into the shape I believed would make me happy. Many people feel this way: *If I just lost fifteen pounds, then I'd be happy. If I could look like that guy, then I'd be happy.* But in the end, no matter what goal I hit, I was always left feeling empty. That's because I had worked really hard to shape the container, but had completely ignored the soul inside of it.

But when you work on your physical and spiritual body simultaneously, through prayer and surrendering to Christ:

- You are more likely to stick with healthier habits.
- You are more appreciative of what you've gained or lost (even if you haven't reached that perfect weight or dress size quite yet).
- You find you have the desire to wake up every day and want to try again, instead of wearily muddling through the motions.
- You find a dependable source of strength to carry you through—and that limitless power comes from Jesus Christ.

IT'S ABOUT PUTTING GOD FIRST— FOREVER AND ALWAYS

At the heart of it, most of us are driven to get in shape to meet others' expectations or approval. Whether we want to become fit to impress our friends, get healthy to appease our doctors, or change our appearance to attract someone we're interested in romantically, we will never be satisfied with the results. As Galatians 1:10 tells us:

Am I now trying to win the favor and approval of men, or of God? Or am I seeking to please someone? If I were still trying to be popular with men, I would not be a bond-servant of Christ.

Even if your goal is simply to look and feel better for yourself, you are probably going to struggle on your own. To stay committed, you need to have a reason to make big changes that is bigger than yourself, one that goes beyond the approval of others or reaching specific numbers on a scale. You need to have a reason that provides a continual source of strength that can carry you not just to the finish line but throughout the rest of your life.

Your reason for changing your lifestyle needs to be growing and developing your relationship with Him.

He Delivers the Strength. When building and strengthening your relationship with God is your primary motivator for changing your lifestyle, He becomes your source of power. During those moments when we are uncomfortable and want to give up, God can rejuvenate us and keep us moving forward. His love is always there for us, giving us the energy, desire, and self-discipline to persevere, especially in times when we don't feel like going any further.

He Offers a New Perspective. Many people already know what healthy habits we should be following. But very few of us make the connection between those habits and how they draw us closer to God. As it turns out, doing things that honor Him—as well as enjoying what He has provided us—can have a positive effect on our physical bodies as well. When you combine faith and fitness, as we will do in this book, you usually find that the changes required to live a healthier life become easier because you *want* to do them—rather than feel you *have* to do them—because these changes bring you closer to God. You recognize that it's not that you *need* to exercise, eat right, and be healthy, but that you *deserve* to exercise, eat right, and be healthy and that these things bring glory to God.

He Fills Every Void. A significant part of most lifestyle programs revolves around removing unhealthy things from your life. (You'll find that in this program as well, by the way.) But you can't expect someone to substitute their old habits for new ones—habits you hope they'll maintain for life—without finding something to fill whatever void is created. But if you strengthen your relationship with God, you quickly discover how He is ready to fill those voids. More important, through a better relationship with Him, you may uncover (and heal) additional voids inside you that you weren't aware of. There may be deep-seated issues behind why you eat or exercise poorly, suffer from low self-esteem, or feel unworthy of being fit and healthy in the first place. You may even discover that the reason you've never been able to make changes is that you never truly believed you could. But remember—with God, all things are possible.

He Walks Beside You. A lot of people don't enjoy a lifestyle program because they don't have a partner. They need somebody working alongside them to push them when they need a push and comfort them when things seem insurmountable. But when you put God first and walk with Him—and allow Him to take this journey with you—you're never alone. Not for one single second. Hebrews 13:5 tells us that He will never leave us nor forsake us. He is always there with us, especially in those moments when we struggle most. Having an undying faith that God is there with us, every step of the way, brings a sense of hope that allows us to reach a little bit further within ourselves than we could ever do on our own.

His Love Knows No Boundaries. Finally, if you feel that you already have a healthy relationship with God, yet living a healthy lifestyle has still escaped you, remember this: I'm not putting your faith in question. In fact, if you're already in the most fantastic place with God, I love that, because that is exactly where you should always be with Him. I know that I also feel that my relationship with God couldn't possibly become any better than it already is. But perhaps you've never considered using your closeness with Him in a way that makes an impact on even more aspects of your life, especially nutrition and exercise. That's what the Seven Sundays program can do; it uses that bond to build upon other areas of your life that you may be struggling with. However, I'm also aware that He is never-ending and that there's always room for improvement in every relationship.

When I talk to those who have been walking with Christ for years or their entire lives, they're usually quick to tell me how He is continually teaching them new things every single day. But when we feel that we have it all together with Him, that sense of ego and pride can prevent us from growing as close as we could be. Because if you don't have a humbled heart, that stops God from coming into those places where we struggle.

It may be as simple as recognizing that when you love someone, you should always be asking yourself, Am I taking this relationship for granted—and are there ways I could help it grow? This journey will not take you away from where you are right now with Him. It's designed to strengthen what you already have and to better your relationship with Him—and to better yourself as a result. It's about realizing that we need to rely on Him in order to move forward.

3

THE PILLARS OF PROMISE

The Seven Sundays program is a faith and fitness regime specifically designed to improve both the spiritual body and the physical body simultaneously by guiding you through a specific set of tasks for six full weeks. But before you begin, because this program involves changing both what you eat and your activity level, my advice is to check with a physician to make sure you're healthy enough to start.

That said, how exactly does it build both the physical and the spiritual at the same time? By focusing on steps that fortify the underpinnings of the Seven Sundays program, which I call the Pillars of Promise.

The three Pillars that lead to a healthy spiritual body are:

Concede (to Christ)
Honor Him (through scripture)
Offer (Making an offering)

The three Pillars that lead to a healthy physical body are:

Sleep
Exercise
Nutrition

When you don't address all six Pillars, you don't connect your physical body with your relationship with God—and that makes it much harder to stay committed to a healthy life. But when you give all six Pillars the same amount of respect and commitment, it fosters a stronger and deeper connection with Him, as well as allowing you to make the changes required to live a healthy, more fulfilled life. That's why throughout the Seven Sundays program, you'll be addressing all of these Pillars of Promise every day.

You may have noticed something about the Pillars of Promise already, and that is how the first letters of each Pillar spell out C.H.O.S.E.N—or *chosen*.

Why *chosen*?

Because it reminds you that each day along your Seven Sundays journey, you'll be asked to make choices, and it's what you choose to do every day that ultimately decides how far you'll walk with Him and eventually succeed with your goals. More important, it's to remind you that God has chosen you, as 2 Thessalonians 2:13 tells us:

> *But we should and are obligated always to give thanks to God for you, believers beloved by the Lord, because God has chosen you from the beginning for salvation through the sanctifying work of the Spirit and by your faith in the truth.*

There are so many people out in the world—so many whom we believe are doing amazing things. If we compare ourselves to them, sometimes it can feel like we just blend in. But God is specific when He says that He has chosen you, and the sheer magnitude of that can change your life.

When I remind myself that I am chosen, I feel unique, special, and loved—and I am reminded that I have a purpose on earth. It keeps alive that special feeling within myself that can sometimes get lost or go unrecognized. That's why, as you run through each Pillar of Promise every day throughout your Seven Sundays journey, you should take a moment and remember how they spell the word *chosen*—to remember that you are too.

———

Throughout the book, you'll see many of my favorite Bible verses that serve as inspiration during the Seven Sundays program. I use the Amplified version of the Bible and cite verses from it each day along your journey. However, you are free to use your own Bible in whatever translation you choose whenever there's a Bible verse mentioned. It won't change your journey in any way; in fact, using whichever version you're most comfortable with will only enhance Seven Sundays for you.

THE PILLARS OF PROMISE DEFINED

So how will you be addressing each of the six Pillars of Promise each day? Here's a look at what you can expect, as well as what you'll achieve:

Concede (to Christ)

The very definition of *concede* is "to surrender"—to admit or acknowledge something that is true. At the start of every morning, before your day begins, you'll set the table by saying a brief prayer surrendering yourself aloud to Him. You'll acknowledge where you are in your journey and what you may need of Him—needs tied into the steps and actions you'll undergo spiritually and physically that day.

It's easy to forget that God needs to comes first. I know that sometimes when my life gets extremely busy, and I feel like I'm being pulled in a thousand directions, I suddenly find myself thinking only about myself and forgetting God. And once that happens, you lose focus and fall off track.

By starting off the day conceding to Christ, you're putting Him at the center of every single day. By surrendering to Him every morning through this acknowledgment, you'll be admitting how much you need Him for the strength to move forward. In surrendering, we recognize that the biggest reason we often fail is that we never concede to Him, and that we will always push ourselves harder for something greater than ourselves.

Finally, this conceding isn't merely something to say once each morning but to repeat throughout the day—as often as you like—whenever you need to remind yourself who you're taking this journey with and for. You can also repeat it at any point when you feel that what I'm asking you to do is awkward, difficult, or impossible. By engaging in this acknowledgment, and by conceding throughout the day, you'll be placing God back in the center, where He belongs, so that you can draw strength through Him during those weakest moments.

Honor Him (through Scripture)

The Bible is His written message to us, and turning to Scripture as often as possible gives us the opportunity to experience so many valuable blessings. God's Word not only guides us through our lives, but it also lifts us and leads us to salvation. And as much as we personally benefit by reading Scripture, it also serves as a way to show reverence to God. It shows how much His Word is appreciated in our lives and how we continually seek the wisdom and guidance He has graciously given us through Scripture.

As you go through this journey, certain moments may be harder than others. For you, it might be the day I ask you to break a particular habit or find the courage to approach others to ask how you can help. That's why it's so important to feed your soul with the right words.

To nourish your spirit along this journey, I will present you with certain scriptures and words of encouragement. These words won't just relate to whatever trials and tribulations you may be undergoing that day; they will also connect with whatever revelations or celebrations may also be a part of it.

I hope that you will meditate on that scripture throughout the day. Try closing your eyes and visualizing it so that every word becomes a part of you, and know that you can continuously return to that scripture for encouragement and a sense of foundation. But most important, realize that these verses are presented to show you that His Word is always connected to our lives. That what was written all those years ago still applies now—and is meant for you.

Offer (Making an Offering)

It doesn't take much to make a big difference in someone else's life. And in serving others, you often make a change in your own life as well. That's why each day, I've suggested a way to give something in His service—an offering in the form of time, love, support, encouragement, effort, or appreciation.

The magic of these offerings is that many will incorporate people whom you love into your journey. In fact, you'll most likely find yourself spending more time with friends, family, and loved ones than ever before throughout the Seven Sundays program. Specific offerings may even expand your base of loved ones by introducing you to people you otherwise may never have had the pleasure of knowing.

Though these offerings are designed to build a healthy spiritual body, you'll probably find that because some may require using a little elbow grease to help out a friend, your church, or your community, you'll find yourself building a healthier physical body as well.

Sleep

We spend a third of our time here on earth asleep (or at least we should be doing that). How we spend that time not only plays a significant part in the overall health of our physical body; it also has an enormous effect on our spiritual body as well.

During sleep, our bodies rebuild themselves at a faster rate, and our immune system releases more T cells, white blood cells that fight viruses, and certain growth hormones to stave off infection.[1] But when you're sleep-deprived, your memory and logical reasoning become impaired, your metabolism slows down (so you burn fewer calories twenty-four/seven), and your body releases more of the stress hormone cortisol. Too much cortisol in your system can disrupt almost all your body's processes (including your immune system and digestive system), and it increases your risk of numerous health conditions, ranging from anxiety and depression to heart disease and weight gain.

But getting enough sleep is equally important for your spirit. The stresses and anxieties our spirits absorb are often due to how we react to the many situations and circumstances we encounter throughout the day. When we're fully rested, we're less apt to be as emotional, and it puts us more in control over those situations and circumstances. It allows us to make better choices because we're thinking with a well-rested mind.

Waking up refreshed will also leave you more alert and more receptive to all the steps throughout the Seven Sundays journey. It will allow you to have plenty of energy and passion to do everything that will soon be required of you so that you're able to draw heavily from those experiences and feel even more fulfilled.

That's why every day throughout Seven Sundays, you'll be given various tips, tricks, and techniques to make you feel more rested, to allow your physical body to recover faster, and to help dissolve any stresses or anxieties that may be keeping your spiritual body from soaring.

Exercise

The exercise portion of Seven Sundays relies on just ten basic moves—five exercises you'll do indoors on certain days, and five you'll do outside on other days. You'll find full descriptions of each exercise at the end of the book, in case you're not familiar with the moves.

It's really important to try to get outdoors on the outdoor days. When you are exercising outside, you won't just be building lean muscle and burning calories. You'll also be spending time with Him, appreciating the glorious gifts He has placed on this earth. That's why you'll be encouraged to exercise outdoors for a minimum of twice weekly. However, if that's not possible on certain days (due to inclement weather or any other reason), you can take your workout indoors.

The program you'll follow will progress from week to week but easily adapts to your current fitness level. You'll perform all the exercises back-to-back with no rest in between. If you find any exercise too difficult, you can opt to try a variation of that exercise that's more *forgiving*. If you find any exercise too easy, you can choose to try a variation of that exercise that's more *aspiring*.

Again, if you're new to exercise or unsure how to do a certain exercise, all the moves are thoroughly explained in the back of the book. I've also taken the time to post instructional videos of all ten moves for your convenience at my website, alecpenix.com.

Nutrition

Seven Sundays isn't a diet book, but you will shed unhealthy weight as you grow closer to God by eating the way He always intended you to eat. In this program, you won't be concerned or counting how many grams of fat or how many calories are in what you're eating, or micromanaging everything that finds its way onto your plate.

Instead, each day you'll follow certain guidelines, as well as learn how specific foods are a direct connection with Him, while others—primarily man-made foods—were never part of God's plan. Instead of counting calories, you'll reflect on what's inside the foods we eat and learn how the right foods will allow you to participate more in life, improve your relationship with your family and friends, build your sense of self-worth, and give you more strength on earth to do His will.

4

THE SEVEN SUNDAYS

And we know that God causes all things to work together
for good for those who love God, to those who are called
according to His plan and purpose.
—ROMANS 8:28

Most lifestyle programs are set out in a week-by-week plan. They might tell you what to do day-to-day, but very few take the time to have you think about what you're about to embark on each day or what they might say to help encourage you along in that exact moment.

With Seven Sundays, every single day is unique and its own journey, and I'm going to walk you through each and every step.

We are now in this together, and I want you to feel special and stay inspired. I never want any feelings of boredom to wash over you, and the way that Seven Sundays is designed, that's one possibility you'll never have to worry about. Here's how it all breaks down:

You'll Begin Your Journey on a Sunday (the First Sunday).

Every day, you'll be instructed on what to do to build upon each of the Pillars of Promise (Conceding, Honoring, Offering, Sleep, Exercise, and Nutrition). Just follow the instructions for each day as best as you can. If you can't manage everything asked of you, that's entirely fine. Just be proud of what you can do and forgive yourself for what you can't.

You'll Rest and Reflect Every Sunday in Between.

Every Sunday, you'll take the time to *recover* (from the week prior), *reflect* (on where you are now along your walk with Him), and *ready* yourself (for what awaits you both physically and spiritually in the week ahead). You won't be exercising on this day, but I hope you will set aside some time to really focus on what happened the previous week and what is to come.

You'll End Your Journey on a Sunday (the Seventh Sunday).

On this final day, you'll reflect on everything you were able to achieve among the Pillars of Promise. But most important, you'll reflect upon your relationship with God and where you stand with Him Seven Sundays later.

———

Even though your journey spans seven Sundays, the program lasts for a total of six weeks, and each week has its own theme, each lasting for seven days, beginning on a Sunday and ending on a Saturday. Each theme also builds upon the last in a way that prepares you for the following week's set of challenges:

- During **Week One**, you'll open your eyes to what has led you to where you are now through a week of *illumination*.
- During **Week Two**, you'll begin to add what's been missing in your life through a week of *elevation*.
- During **Week Three**, you'll remove what is toxic to your physical and spiritual bodies through a week of *purification*.
- During **Week Four**, you'll explore how to modify what you've learned through a week of *adaptation*.
- During **Week Five**, you'll intensify your bond with Him through a week of *glorification*.
- During **Week Six**, you'll commit yourself fully to Him through a week of *dedication*.

WHY BEGIN THE PROGRAM ON A DAY OF WORSHIP?

Most lifestyle programs start on a Monday, and even when they don't specify a day to begin, many people prefer Mondays because it allows them one last hurrah over the weekend before taking things seriously. And when it comes to Sundays, well—that day is usually flagged as a day off, either because it's the Lord's day or simply as a day to rest from all the hard work performed throughout the week. A day of rest is a good thing—that's how the Lord designed it, after all. But for some people, Sundays can become a step backward when it comes to health and fitness because they leave many people with little direction beyond *rest*. Lack of a purpose makes it that much easier to step off the path and either cheat or quit.

But with this regime, Sundays are the most important days of the program. That's because you'll not only spend Sundays allowing your body to heal through proper rest and recovery, but you'll also use these days to both reflect on—and find direction in—the program on a day when we typically feel the most connected to Him.

WHAT IF I ALREADY FOLLOW A DAILY DEVOTIONAL?

The ideas and scriptures within the Seven Sundays program are not meant to be a replacement for what you may already follow. What I share with you each day is only meant to enlighten and encourage you along your journey. Know that you're always free to explore other scriptures along the way, especially if you find certain verses more beneficial in certain moments when you need motivation or clarity.

DO I HAVE TO DO EVERYTHING YOU SUGGEST?

That is entirely up to you. This journey is, first and foremost, about strengthening *your* relationship with God. How far you're able to grow with Him depends on what *you're* willing to put into Seven Sundays. But just as God is forgiving, you should forgive yourself if you're not able to follow every step of the way.

I'm certain there might be a few changes that could be too difficult to incorporate or master—for now at least. I also understand there may be an offering or two that might either make you feel uncomfortable or could be impossible to pull off on a particular day. Ideally, I hope that you do it all because every step serves a higher purpose, and I don't want you to miss out on what's achievable when you follow every step along this journey with Him. So just try your best. Because no matter what, He will reward you for what you put forth.

Seven Sundays isn't just about losing pounds—it's about encountering more of a purpose in your life. It's about looking at how you can influence your friends, your family, others in your community—and yes, even the world—through your actions and reactions. It's not about *having* to look better for that class reunion to make former classmates jealous; it's about *wanting* to show a better side of yourself and possibly inspire others. It's a much broader picture than just staring in the mirror and finally loving what you see. It's about being proud of the person staring back and knowing they are genuinely happy, never alone, and always loved.

He's waiting for you—now let's begin.

PART TWO

The Seven Sundays Journey

For all the peoples walk each in the name of his god. As for us, we shall walk in the name of the Lord our God forever and ever.
—MICAH 4:5

DAY 1 (SUNDAY)

THE FIRST SUNDAY

The Week of Illumination (Days 1 through 7)

During this first week, you will not be asked to make any changes to your sleep habits, exercise regime, or diet. Instead these first seven days are about illumination, a time when your goal is to enlighten yourself . . . well, about yourself!

On this day, throughout this day, ask yourself: What made me pick up this book in the first place? Where do I want to see change in my life? Am I hoping to see a difference in the mirror or a difference in myself—or both? Where do I feel like I'm struggling the most? Am I happy with where I'm at physically or spiritually? Do I favor one at the expense of the other? What are the areas of my life in which I am not trusting God?

As you spend time with Him today, let the Holy Spirit come through, be honest with both the Lord and yourself, and remind yourself about the areas of your life—physically and spiritually—in which you would like to see growth.

Concede

God, I need to be shown what it is to be reborn again. I need newness and a fresh outlook with myself and toward the journey ahead. I ask that You show me the areas that may be blocking me from moving forward in life. I ask You for a fresh start. Thank You, Father. Amen.

Honor

As you embark on this journey, you may be concerned that your past will prevent you from staying true to the present and making a difference in your future. That is why I like to consider 2 Corinthians 5:17 on this very first day:

> *Therefore if anyone is in Christ, he is a new creature; the old things have passed away. Behold, new things have come.*

This verse speaks about how we are all new creatures through Him. It's about having a fresh beginning and creating new habits for ourselves. It's about how we have the strength within us to change our own life and detach ourselves from our failures and bad choices of the past.

Maybe you've tried other programs before. In fact, I'm certain you have. But focusing on past mistakes and failure can keep the best of us from moving forward. That's why surrendering to the process—and letting God take the reins—is so crucial on this first day. This journey is about letting your past fade away to allow yourself to be open to new things. No matter how far you've already come in your life up to this point, remind yourself that you're now in the process of creating something new starting today. And remember that, through Him, you are always reborn.

Offer

Today is about offering your hand to a good cause—guided by what the Lord needs that day. So when you attend church today, ask how you can serve. It's a rare church that isn't looking for volunteers for one thing or another, and I suspect that if you're willing to offer yourself, you'll find a way to serve the body of Christ. For just as we must give ourselves over to God, we must give ourselves over to the church—without any Hope of glory—to help both our congregation and our community.

Your offering doesn't have to be huge; just give what you're able to. If you ask and find that they don't have any needs at the moment, that's fine—the mere intention of giving yourself to the church is an offering in itself.

What you do for the church isn't of consequence either. Whether it's baking something for a committee meeting, sorting through donated clothing, volunteering as an usher, or cleaning up after a function, it's all service to the Lord. It is about not waiting to be asked, but instead finding where you are needed.

If you don't go to church that often (or belong to one), don't let that stop you from doing what you can. Let the Holy Spirit guide you, and visit whatever church feels right to you; then ask to speak to someone about how you can help. Again, it doesn't matter if you're a regular church attendee—what matters is that you're attending *a* church on this day.

Sleep

Throughout this week, you'll be asked to assess certain things that may be preventing you from resting correctly. But today I only ask that you ponder how you felt this morning when you woke up.

- Was it a struggle, or did you spring out of bed?
- Did you feel as if you needed more sleep, or would resting longer have felt like a waste of your morning?
- Were specific places on your body achy, particularly in neck, back, arms, or shoulders?
- Was there something on your mind the night before that is still on your mind this morning?

For now, don't question *why* you may feel a certain way upon waking. Instead I only wish you to remind yourself of *what* you felt.

Exercise

During this first week, you won't be performing any specific exercises. However, I will ask you to walk with Him on certain days. The duration of each of these Worship Walks will gradually build from thirty minutes to sixty minutes in length. That's why today I want you to prepare ahead of time by making sure you have a proper pair of walking shoes, as well as a few places in mind to walk.

If one of your ambitions for taking part in the Seven Sundays program is weight loss, then imagine your goals regarding weight loss, but be realistic about your expectations. Often we set ourselves up for failure with fitness because we place our hopes at a height that is physically impossible to reach safely. What you must remind yourself is that the healthiest approach for your body is to experience a loss of one to two pounds per week—and that's all.

Depending on how many changes you make along your journey, especially with nutrition, you may lose a little more. But for now, acknowledge this number, and understand that losing weight at a pace of more than two pounds a week only means you're most likely losing water through dehydration or burning off valuable lean muscle tissue, not the body fat you're hoping to shed. It also means you're most likely pushing your body past a healthy point by either eating far less than your body needs or doing too much exercise (which can lead to overtraining and increase your risk of getting sick or injured). None of these outcomes are things you want to experience if being in the best shape (and health) possible are part of your goals.

Nutrition

Over the course of this first week, you won't be asked to change a thing about your diet. Instead your only goal will be to become more aware of what you eat and drink, how often you eat, what's in the foods you eat and drink, and finally, what you hope to achieve through attention to your nutritional habits.

Every few days, you'll be asked to try something new that will open your eyes to the foods around you—and what you expect from your diet. To accomplish this, the only thing you'll need to prepare for the upcoming week will be a small journal to write in after each meal or snack.

But before you take this walk, treat yourself to something food-based today that brings you delight. In other words, give in to your guilty pleasure. Maybe that means Sunday brunch with friends or indulging in dessert after dinner.

This may be the exact opposite of what you would expect on Day 1 of any lifestyle program, but there are several reasons why I don't mind if you give in to a good meal.

When you allow yourself this "reward," don't just devour it. Instead, truly concentrate on what about that meal or treat is bringing you joy. As you eat, think about what it is that is ultimately satisfying.

- Is it the taste? If so, then perhaps there are other ways you could satisfy that craving with a healthier food that shares the same flavor.

- Is it that it's out of your routine? If so, might it be possible to start a new routine using more nutritious foods?
- Does it trigger a happy memory, such as when you were a child or at a more joyous time in your life? If so, are there other non-food activities that might have the same effect?
- Is it the social aspect? If so, can you have the same moment with friends and family without the need to attach food to it?

You may come to realize that what you've chosen as your "guilty pleasure" was picked for a reason that may be valid, but that doesn't mean it has to be unhealthy. You may come to realize that it's not the ingredients of the foods you're eating, but the environment and emotions connected with our "cheat meals" that make them hard to resist.

DAY 2 (MONDAY)

Concede

Father, I ask that Your hand open up to me today as a gesture of Your graciousness. I've been humbled, and I know it's only Your grace that can save me now. Allow me to experience Your hand at work in my life, so that I may know You are here by my side. Thank You, Father, Amen.

Honor

Although it's only the second day of your journey, what's important to remember is that you're giving God the reins and allowing Him to take authority over your life. That's what makes Acts 7:49–50 a compelling message to meditate upon today:

> *"Heaven is My throne, and the earth is the footstool for My feet; what kind of house will you build for Me?" says the Lord, "or what place is there for My rest? Was it not My hand that made all these things?"*

These scriptures represent the authority of God, and how His hand is placed on our lives and directs it. One of the steps you'll be taking today is connected to this idea. Today you'll be writing down what you eat. It's a step not to be taken lightly because it is by your hand that you will be evaluating your actions to change them for the better. You'll have to be honest in your records, because you can't allow God to take authority over your life if you're not entirely authentic. So bring to this day, as with every day, complete honesty, and share with Him all your actions—and know that you're not being judged.

Offer

On this second day, all I ask is that you smile as often as possible, for as long as possible, even if you don't necessarily feel happy at the moment.

A smile is simple. It doesn't take any effort or thought, and yet this act may be one of the most powerful offerings you will make throughout the Seven Sundays journey. It's also one of the few offerings that I insist you master not just today, but on every day along your journey. But on this day, pay close attention to the power that comes from wearing a smile.

We carry our emotions forward. We share how we feel, and who we are, with others we come in contact with all day long, even before we get to say a single word.

A smile is inviting and makes others want to be a part of that happiness. Smiling tells others that you're friendly and ready to connect, and a smile makes you seem like a person whom others will want to connect with. When you don't smile, you may be passing up opportunities to connect merely because your face creates a closed door that's locked tight. It can make you seem less approachable and preoccupied in a way that might cause others to leave you alone.

A smile is also infectious. When we smile, others around us tend to do the same. But, more important, smiling can also change their attitude at the same time, giving them more hope and happiness at a time when they may need it most.

I will admit that I've had a handful of clients reveal how difficult this simple task can sometimes be, particularly on days when they thought they had nothing to smile about. And maybe that's you today—or you may expect it to be you eventually throughout Seven Sundays. When that's the case, then consider this:

- Do you have family members who love you? Are there others in your life who care about you?
- Are you in good health? Are those close to you in good health?
- Have you experienced harder times than you're presently going through right now?
- If I asked you to recall something from your past that made you happy, what would it be?

When you take a moment to reflect, there are always people, memories, or circumstances in our lives that make us feel joyful and blessed. Realize that you still have at least one reason—and I'm confident many reasons—to smile all day long. It's all about having the right perspective and appreciating the blessing that God has already given you, rather than focusing on what you feel is missing in your life at this moment.

Sleep

Bringing ourselves to a better place of rest begins with the smallest of steps. The most obvious is merely being aware of how long we allow ourselves to rest in the first place. So this morning your only task is to count back from the time you woke up until the time you went to bed—and count the hours in between.

The right number of hours varies by person, but most experts agree that we need between seven and nine hours. Once you know how long you've slept, reduce that number by about an hour. Why? Research has shown that most people typically misjudge how much they sleep, adding an average of forty-eight minutes more than they actually achieved.[1]

If your number is less than seven, you don't have to change anything yet. We'll work on that as we move forward, and along this journey, you'll absorb many things that will make getting more sleep an easier task. For now, simply remind yourself that the goal of sleep is to wake up feeling refreshed. If you feel as if you could have spent more time in bed, you're going against how God has meant your body to function and recover.

Exercise

On this day, you'll walk side by side with God for thirty minutes in what I call a Worship Walk. Find somewhere outdoors, preferably a spot that allows you to take in as many of His wonders as possible—and just walk with Him.

When I say "walk with God," some people have a hard time visualizing what I mean. That's because that walk is different for everyone. Essentially, what I mean by this is simple: Just walk, and as you do, imagine that He is walking right alongside you, because He is, every single moment of our lives. As you go, I want you to think about Him every step of the way. For some people, praying as they pace helps keep them focused on God. For others, it's observing all His wonders around them and just marveling at what He's created here on earth for us. And for others, it can mean simply opening your heart and allowing God to speak to you.

I don't want you thinking about the fact that you're exercising, because your spirit should be in a different place. These Worship Walks aren't merely about conditioning your muscles and keeping your heart healthy; they are about being conscious of God. They are meant to connect your movement to a spiritual level. But here's what's interesting: when you put yourself in a different place spiritually, it can change the dynamic of exercise for you.

You see, when we work out, we can be more in tune with our bodies. We feel our endorphins rising, our pulse quickening, our blood pumping, and our muscles working collectively—and that puts us in a fantastic place to hear from God. As we focus, through exercise, on our body—the vessel He chose for us—we are reminded of how marvelously designed we really are. How He intended our bodies to respond to resistance in a way that naturally adapts and improves if we stick with it. And as you watch your body acclimate and progress throughout Seven Sundays, remind yourself that your spirit is equally adaptable—a point that many of us never ponder. But it is if you are both patient and persistent.

Do I Need Any Special Clothing or Equipment?

Not beyond the walking shoes I recommended that you wear on Sunday. In terms of clothing, just put on what makes sense and what's most comfortable. You don't need to invest in any equipment, such as a pedometer, exercise tracker, or anything that monitors your fitness. In fact, if you're paying less attention to these small details, you'll be able to remain more focused on just appreciating your time with Him.

Do I Have to Walk?

So long as you move with Him for thirty minutes, you can maintain any pace you wish. If you're able to jog or run for that length of time, go for it, so long as a faster pace doesn't distract you from being with Him at that moment.

Can I Listen to Music?

Yes, if it's something that still allows God to speak to you at this moment. My worship runs change every single day. Sometimes I listen to sermons as I run, while other days I may listen to worship music. But most days, I prefer no distractions. I want to hear myself breathe, listen to nature around me, and be able to connect with the thoughts that come through my head during those moments. The choice is up to you.

What if It's Rainy, Too Hot, or Too Cold?

If the weather isn't agreeable, you can bring your workout inside and walk on a treadmill, if you have access to one. If not, you can always walk in place or pace around your house, so long as you aren't distracted by other things. However, I encourage you (when possible) to try and figure out a way to head outside because otherwise you'll be missing out on observing and surrounding yourself with nature. If it's raining, then think about investing in some rain gear that will help you stay dry. If it's too hot, then plan your walks either early or late in the day when the sun isn't at its highest. Finally, if it's too cold, then dress appropriately and remember that you are blessed to have the means to do so. Let the changing weather serve not as an obstacle, but as both a test to triumph over and a reminder of what an amazing place He has given us to live.

What if I Live in a City?

If you're somewhere more urban, and getting to a park or a place that puts you more in touch with nature isn't possible, then recognize that God is all around us, even in the midst of a bustling city. As you walk, try to find nature at every turn. You might just have to pay a little more attention to hear the birds singing. Notice the lone tree growing alongside a busy street. Casually glance up at the sky and observe the clouds passing by, or let yourself really enjoy the sun shining on your face. Even in the most metropolitan of areas, you'll find that He is all around us. It just takes a little awareness to notice.

What if I Can't Do Thirty Minutes Straight, Either Due to My Current Fitness Level or Lack of Time?

The exercise portion of Seven Sundays is entirely adaptable. Even the strength-training movements you'll be learning soon are easily modifiable according to your current fitness level. If you find that walking for thirty minutes is difficult, you may break up your Worship Walk into two fifteen-minute walks or three ten-minute walks instead. Ideally, I would prefer your workout to be one, long continuous walk, because the longer we speak with someone, the more in-depth that conversation typically is. Each Worship Walk is technically a conversation with God, so by breaking up your workout, you're interrupting that conversation in a way that may prevent a deeper dive with Him. However, dividing up your routine also means you'll have more opportunities to walk with Him during the day, so if that's more comfortable for you, then know you won't be sacrificing anything using that approach. The most important thing is to walk with Him for thirty minutes.

Nutrition

Today is all about bringing consciousness to what you're eating. To do that, you'll keep a log of everything you eat.

It's easy to fudge the facts when you're doing this. Sometimes we are afraid to admit what we're really putting into our bodies. Remember, Seven Sundays is a program built entirely on honesty, and the only person you're being dishonest with is yourself—because this log is for no one *but* yourself. You deserve more than that. It's better to be transparent than less forthcoming. Besides, this is only meant as a guide to show you how much your diet is evolving as you move through Seven Sundays.

How you perform this task is up to you. When working with clients, I have them use an app that tracks the foods they're eating. But for this task, you don't have to be as specific. If you prefer:

Jot down each meal or snack on a piece of paper or in a journal. Make sure you write the time, as well as the size of each item. You don't need to get a food scale; doing this can be as simple as estimating the volume by writing "a fistful of berries" or "a hand-sized piece of fish."

Skip writing altogether, and instead take a picture of each meal and snack with your phone. Each picture will be time-stamped, so you'll know the size of your portions and when you consumed them. That goes for every beverage as well, so if you have more than one, make sure you snap a shot of every glass, cup, or mug.

Finally, don't worry if you're documenting some dietary choices that you're not proud of. The more honest you are now, the more satisfied you'll be later on. It's about taking ownership of all your actions so that every Sunday you'll begin to take pride when you compare and contrast with what you've eaten the week before.

DAY 3 (TUESDAY)

Concede

Father, I ask that You hold me a little closer today. I want to become familiar with Your comfort and knowing that You will never leave me nor forsake me. I surrender with all my heart, my mind, my soul, and my strength so that You can come and do Your work. Thank You, Father. Amen.

Honor

It's comforting to know that there's someone you can turn to. Whether it's your parents or a good friend, your partner or your children, there are certain people who bring comfort just because you know they'll always be there for you. That's why today you'll focus on one single scripture: Deuteronomy 31:8.

> *It is the Lord who goes before you; He will be with you. He will not fail you or abandon you. Do not fear or be dismayed.*

What I love about this verse is that not only does it exemplify the point that you're never alone, but it reminds you that it's the Lord that goes before you. It's akin to holding a parent's hand and having them assure you that you're safe as they take you forward.

That is the mind-set I would like you to retain today and through-out your journey because it's one of the pieces most lifestyle programs never focus on. It's easy to be excited early on when starting a program, but a few days in, that's when the changes you've begun to make in your life start to take effect. That may mean a little muscle soreness or realizing that soon you may not be able to enjoy certain foods. It could be realizing that you now have to begin taking time out of your day to accomplish things you never had to before. In other words, you may quickly find yourself thrown slightly out of your comfort zone. And it's during these times that the excitement you initially felt begins to wane.

But God's with you—and He has your hand. So if things ever feel difficult along the way, instead of focusing on the discomfort of specific changes, focus on the comfort that comes from knowing He never fails us.

Offer

The words *comfort food* are typically associated with the unhealthy fare some people turn to as a source of security when they feel sad, anxious, sick, or upset. But on this day, the term will have a new meaning for you. Instead bring someone food—whether it's a family member, a friend, or even a perfect stranger—to comfort them with care.

Food is a powerful tool for breaking down people's walls. Whether you're sitting down to dinner or stepping out for lunch with someone, the act of eating socially can create a very relaxing atmosphere that allows others to share emotions and feelings more easily than when they are asked, "What's wrong?" So, on this day, prepare or purchase a meal to share with someone who may be—or seems to be—struggling with something in their life.

Ideally, I would encourage you to make the food as healthy as possible, but it doesn't have to be. If you don't think you'll be able to connect with this person easily, then try to remember that this meal is about them. It's about making them more receptive to sitting down and connecting with someone who cares about them. It's not about bringing them a meal as much as it is an opportunity to talk and bond with someone.

Final note: Don't expect success when you bring them comfort. Truth be told, you may not see any change within the person or even get a thank-you. Just remind yourself that this offering is unconditional and isn't about the outcome. It's strictly about the effort.

Sleep

Today ask yourself: When was the last time I washed my bedsheets?

Some people may find this question odd, and I understand that. But I ask it not to make a judgment or for the sake of cleanliness or comfort. I ask out of concern for your health. According to the National Sleep Foundation, roughly three out of four people say they enjoyed a more comfortable night's sleep when their sheets had a fresh, clean scent.[1] More important, unclean sheets contain bacteria that can cause health issues ranging from allergies to pneumonia.

That said, I'd like to ask you to take the time to wash your sheets at least once weekly in hot water, then dry them on low heat (so they don't shrink). Even though this was a week meant to simply illuminate (and not necessarily take action), this vital step is one that simply cannot be reserved for later—and it may play a huge role in how well you adapt to other changes to your sleeping habits further along in the journey.

Exercise

On this day, you'll continue to walk side by side with God. But instead of spending only thirty minutes, add ten more and walk with

Him for forty minutes. Again, as I recommended on Day 2, if this amount of time is difficult, you may divide up that time into several smaller Worship Walks, but I encourage taking one continuous walk with Him.

However, if going from thirty to forty minutes seems too difficult physically, take a look at a few things:

- Was the terrain you walked on yesterday a steeper grade? If so, try to find a flatter surface today.
- What type of pace are you keeping? You may be pushing yourself harder than you have to. Remember, this isn't a race—it's a walk with God. It's a journey that's about spending time with him, not about how hard you sweat as you go.
- Are you maintaining proper form as you walk? Poor posture can cause certain muscles to tire out before they should, so make sure you stand up straight as you walk, pull your stomach in, and keep your head up (eyes facing forward). Your heel should always hit the ground first; roll your foot from heel to toe, and then push off with your toes at the end of each step.

Nutrition

You'll continue to log your food today, but before you begin, take a moment to contemplate anything you may have encountered yesterday when you introduced food journaling into your routine:

- Were there any moments when you found it difficult?
- Is using your phone more comfortable for you than relying on a small journal or tablet?
- Did you feel self-conscious recording what you consumed around other people?

- Have you been completely honest with everything you've written down? If so, then be proud. If not, take pride in being honest with yourself; then simply try to do better today.

If any of these questions revealed inevitable obstacles along the way, think about how you might remove those challenges today—and every day moving forward. It's all about becoming more comfortable with the process of logging and imagining ways that can make the process more comfortable for you.

DAY 4 (WEDNESDAY)

Concede

Lord, fears hold me back. The truth is, I don't know how to deal with it. I ask that You give me the strength to overcome my fears. Not a strength that comes from my own flesh and bones, but a deeper strength that comes from Your love. I want to experience how Your love can cast away all my fears. Thank You, Father. Amen.

Honor

This day is all about overcoming fear, which is what makes 1 John 4:18 the ideal verse to consider today:

> *There is no fear in love. But perfect love drives out fear, because fear involves punishment, so the one who is afraid is not perfected in love.*

Starting anything new can be a challenge, and it's natural to have self-doubt or be nervous about what others might think of us, especially when we are trying something that really puts us out there. After all, people are going to notice that you're trying to change and doing something different with Seven Sundays. Will they question what you're doing? Will they believe in what you're doing?

Whenever we start something new, we may begin eager and excited, but usually when we're a few days in, we start to realize what it is we've taken on. And that's when fear can set in. The fear of failure. The fear of not being strong enough to stay the course. The fear of what might change in our lives that we may not be prepared for. The fear of embarking on something new that may not deliver in the end.

Once the excitement wears off and the hard work begins, we may feel the need to pull back out of fear. But this moment is a blessing in disguise because it's an opportunity to test your faith. If you're able to overcome your fears, you'll remember it not as a day when you failed, but as a day when you flourished.

I chose this verse because it gives a different perspective on fear and how it can be overcome. The reaction most people have when it comes to fear is either to run from it or push through it using sheer will. But running from fear gets us nowhere, while pushing against our fears can sometimes cause us to fall as a result.

What we really need to face our fears with is God's love.

Love casts out all fear, and it's those who don't understand the true capacity of God's love that tend to be overcome by fear most often. So remind yourself what this journey is all about—becoming closer to God—so there's never any reason to fear. For His inexhaustible love is with you always, ready to cast away any and all fears that may come your way. What are you afraid of on this journey? Spend some time thinking and praying about that now.

Offer

Today you'll serve in some way that makes you fearful. It doesn't have to be something that evokes genuine fear, but merely a task that takes you out of your natural element. For example, if you're the shy type, it may be asking you to be the greeter at church this Sunday. It might be helping someone with a task you may not feel qualified to do. It could even be finding the strength to ask for help with something you've been putting off but have been afraid to take on by yourself. It just needs to be something that you know serves Him but requires overcoming your nerves to do it.

What's remarkable is that sometimes we come to find that what scares us may actually be our calling. At other times, facing our fears to help others can help us minimize or remove that fear from that point forward. But until you step out of your element, you'll never know what is truly inside you and what you're capable of.

If you're not certain what task to take on, wait for that moment to come. There is always a moment during each day when you could do His work but choose not to for a particular reason. When that moment arrives, prove to yourself what you're capable of because you have God at your side.

Sleep

The way we position ourselves as we go to bed—as well as the position in which we wake up in the morning—is often an indicator of the posture our bodies most likely maintain as we sleep.

Think about the last time you sat with poor posture for a few hours, such as on a long flight or at your desk. How did your body feel afterward? Think about how *not* moving a muscle can cause pain and discomfort. In fact, poor body positioning at night can lead to headaches, back and neck pain, heartburn, fatigue, sleep apnea, muscle cramping, and circulation issues, among other potential health issues.

Starting today, be conscious of certain things throughout this journey:

- What position do you relax into in order to fall asleep?
- What position do you find yourself in when you wake up?
- Are certain of your body parts feeling stiffer or more painful

in the morning—body parts that weren't as stiff or achy before bedtime?

Keep a mental note of these things throughout the journey because you'll be implementing certain techniques and making slight adjustments that may affect the answers to these questions by the end of Seven Sundays.

Exercise

Today you won't be exercising but instead allowing your body to rest and heal from exercise. I call such a day an Acknowledge-Pray-Rest Day; it's a day to not only avoid activity so your body can recover, but also to acknowledge everything you've achieved over the last few days with your workouts.

For some people, a day off from exercise is a welcome change. But for others, particularly those who think you have to exercise every day to see change, taking time off can cause worry. Just know that these Acknowledge-Pray-Rest Days are in place to prevent you from pushing yourself too hard. It's through rest that we grow, and by resting today, you'll be readying your body—both physically and spiritually—to be active tomorrow.

When you work out, you're essentially putting your body through a type of stress that breaks down muscle tissue and burns through glycogen (the carbohydrates stored in your muscles that your body also turns to for energy during exercise) in addition to stored fat. But after your workout is over, that's when the real work begins, as your body begins to repair itself, rebalancing the oxygen levels in your blood, replacing glycogen in your muscles, and rebuilding muscle tissue. Why? So you're not only ready to exercise again a day or so later, but so you come back to your workouts a little fitter and stronger.

On these days, I don't merely want you to recover, but to contemplate how you could improve your next exercise session. It's about really taking a hard look at what might be preventing you from establishing a higher bond with God. That said, on any Acknowledge-Pray-Rest Day throughout the journey, consider the following and make changes accordingly:

- Was there anything that distracted you along the way? If so, you may want to consider how to remove those distractions.
- Did you find it too difficult? If that's a yes, consider some of the options to make the workout more forgiving.
- Could I use a change of scenery? Trust your heart. I find that some people prefer familiarity and achieve a greater closeness with God by walking the same terrain over and over again. For others, changing things around each time works best to prevent boredom and help them appreciate more of God's work around them.

Nutrition

My wish for you is to have healthy dietary expectations that never lead you to failure. So today your only task is to figure out a nutritional goal for yourself.

It should be measurable. Simply saying I want to eat healthier or I want to feel better is a difficult goal to define. Instead try being more specific, such as deciding you want to add ten healthier foods into your diet.

It should be achievable. Expecting to lose forty to fifty pounds is a terrific goal, but trying to lose that much in the space of Seven Sundays just isn't realistic, nor is it healthy. As noted above for Day 1, losing one to two pounds a week is a normal pace, and it is achievable if you remain true to both the diet and exercise portions of the Seven Sundays program. So if losing weight is one of your goals, a more realistic number to consider would be about six to twelve pounds.

It should be honorable. What are your intentions for eating healthier? Is it only to look good, or is it so you can be more active with your family, live longer, or lead by example? The fact remains: the more altruistic your goal, the more strength you'll find within yourself to stick to and achieve that goal.

DAY 5 (THURSDAY)

Concede

Father, I know that You love me, and I love You, but what I need help with is how to love myself. Show me how beautifully made I am and how to see myself through Your eyes. I am Your clay, and You are the potter. Mold me into a person that I'm proud to be. Thank You, Father. Amen.

Honor

A great set of verses to ponder, declare, and confess throughout this day is Psalm 139:13–15:

> *For You formed my innermost parts;*
> *You knit me in my mother's womb.*
> *I will give thanks and praise to You, for I am*
> *fearfully and wonderfully made;*
> *Wonderful are Your works,*
> *And my soul knows it very well.*
> *My frame was not hidden from You,*
> *When I was being formed in secret,*

And intricately and skillfully formed in the depths of the earth.

Many times, we either forget or fail to comprehend the depth of love that God has for us. Worse still, we may doubt His love because we don't always love ourselves. Whatever the case may be, when we don't meet God halfway, we can miss many of the blessings He presents us along the way.

The reason I enjoy these verses is that David is explaining how beautifully made we are. We are reminded that we're all created in God's image, and each of us is a woven masterpiece. Sometimes we have distractions in our lives merely because we don't have enough respect for ourselves to get rid of those distractions.

Whether you struggle with loving yourself or not, remain aware that you're chosen by Him, that He loves you, that you're wonderfully made, and that God doesn't make mistakes. Once you have a love for yourself—the same love He has for you—you begin to respect yourself enough to do whatever it takes to make the healthiest choices for yourself.

Offer

Love and trust are part of the same family. When we choose to confide in someone, what we are technically doing is building a relationship by forging a bond with that other person. But what we're also doing is showing that person that they are seen and appreciated as someone dependable and trustworthy.

By sharing something personal about yourself with someone—which is precisely your offering today—you not only strengthen your relationship with that person, but you're showing that you love them and know they will be there for you.

I know some people may not like to speak about their finances, family issues, or other personal problems. So instead of thinking of turmoil to share, think about turnarounds instead. In the Christian community, our testimony is very important, so a great starting place can be how God has worked in your life. It might be talking about how you were in a bad place in your life—a time when everything seemed to be working against you—and God opened a door for you. If you wish, make what you share a victory, about how God brought you out of a less fortunate situation and put you in a place that is fruitful.

The beauty of this offering is that it may also open a door. Often others wish they could share with us, and may see us as trustworthy, but cannot find it within themselves to start the conversation. But putting yourself out there sometimes gives others the courage to do the same. It also makes us remember, through God's love, how far we've risen above that low place we once found ourselves in.

If you're not sure who to speak to, allow yourself to be led by the Holy Spirit and trust that It will reveal somebody on that day whom you should talk with and confide in. It might be noticing someone's body language or noticing that someone who typically walks in with a smile doesn't seem to have one that day. If you simply remain aware and observe your friends, your family, your coworkers, members of your congregation—or anyone you come in contact with during the day—the Holy Spirit will reveal someone going through something in that moment.

You could go up to them and say something as simple as, "I hope you're doing okay today. A while back, I was going through something, and God brought me through it. If there's anything going on that you'd like to talk about, just know that I'm here. And if not, just know that God has you." This simple gesture alone brings acknowledgment that someone does see them and reminds them that God is with them. It's confirmation that even in their darkest days, God is still with them.

Sleep

Today think strategically about the sheets and blankets you use on your bed. What keeps you warm at night is surrounding you for roughly a third of your day, so ask yourself the following questions regarding your bedding:

- Do you find yourself waking up sweaty? If it's too difficult to simply throw off a sheet or two (because your partner may not appreciate it), you may want to consider choosing sheets made from natural fibers like cotton and bamboo or from high-tech wicking fabrics that pull sweat away from your skin.
- How old is your bedding? The more you wash it, the more worn (and less comfy) your bedding can become. If it's more than two years old, you may want to consider something new and fresh.
- Does your bedding have a certain amount of weight to it? Using either a weighted blanket or layering several blankets on top of yourself can mimic a form of deep-touch therapy that may ease anxiety and encourage sleep in a way similar to swaddling an infant. It's not just that a heavier blanket feels like a big, comforting hug; it also actually helps to increase the release of serotonin and relaxes your nervous system, leaving you feeling much calmer and sleepier as a result.

Exercise

On this day, you'll once again walk with God, this time for fifty minutes instead of forty minutes. Again, as I recommended on Day 2, if this amount of time is difficult, you may divide it up into several smaller Worship Walks, but I encourage taking one continuous walk with Him.

Because this is also the first day back after an Acknowledge-Pray-Rest Day, take notice of how you feel physically and spiritually after taking that time to recover. Listening to what your body is trying to tell you after resting is something many people never bother to explore. Ask yourself:

- Do I feel refreshed? Your body should have rested enough so that you feel ready for another day of activity.
- Do I feel a little sore? Your muscles should be slightly sore to some degree, which lets you know that you're accomplishing what you're hoping to do, which is to challenge and strengthen them through physical activity. That slight discomfort means you're working specific muscles that typically don't receive as much attention— and that's a good thing. As long as you aren't feeling any sharp pains, you're merely experiencing normal muscle soreness.

Nutrition

On this day, you'll continue to implement what you've been asked to do throughout this week of illumination: logging your food, as well as reminding yourself of your nutritional goal. If you couldn't decide on a nutritional goal yesterday, then take the time today to do so.

Also, ask yourself if the goal you had yesterday is still your goal today. It's entirely natural for our goals to change, so just be certain that the goal you chose on Day 4 is still top of mind today and wasn't chosen out of haste. If it's still the same, odds are it's a goal you'll continue to focus on, which will make it easier to gauge how much progress you've made moving toward that goal. If it's not, then dig deep and allow yourself more time to find that goal for yourself.

DAY 6 (FRIDAY)

Concede

Father, I thank You for supplying me with everything I need to succeed today. I hereby give all my bad habits over to You. I take authority over my temple; my fleshly temptations will no longer have power over me. Today I only take in things that You desire for me to take in. Thank You, Father. Amen.

Honor

Genesis 1:29–31 reveals:

> So God said, "Behold, I have given you every plant yielding seed that is on the surface of the entire earth, and every tree which has fruit yielding seed; it shall be food for you; and to all the animals on the earth and to every bird of the air and to everything that moves on the ground—to everything in which there is the breath of life—I have given every green plant for food"; and it was so. God saw everything that He had made, and behold, it was very good and He validated it completely. And there was evening and there was morning, a sixth day.

These three verses remind us how everything we have here on earth is because of God—and that He is the creator of all things. On this day, keeping that thought in your heart is crucial, because as you'll come to see, from today on, you'll be trying to look at what you eat from the proper perspective.

Offer

My hope is that you already have a dynamic prayer life in place, which (trust me) will grow even further throughout your journey. And if that's not the case right now, as you move through Seven Sundays, that will be just one of many things that will improve to help you forge a more prosperous relationship with Him. But on this day, commit to pray for someone or an organization that's not necessarily in need but provides for others.

Prayer is a way of giving to somebody. When most people think of giving to others, their minds move to the physical, such as gifts, donations, or monetary gestures. But prayer itself as a potent tool that we can offer others because it's a way of providing for someone spiritually.

Often we reserve prayer for the ones we love and those who need our prayer, which is entirely honorable. But we sometimes forget those that we "believe" may not necessarily be struggling—individuals we may not even know—but are providing for others and performing the Lord's work. But I feel like most people are wrestling with something, even though they may not be showing it outwardly. So today you will pray for someone who is doing good in the world. Offer your spiritual support, and ask the Spirit to reveal whom to pray for.

Sleep

Before you lie down to sleep tonight, reflect on what you're wearing to bed. As it turns out, how you dress for sleep may have a major effect on how quickly you drift off—as well as the quality of your sleep throughout the night. For example, one recent piece of research found that sleep onset latency (the length of time it takes to shift from being fully awake to asleep) is significantly shortened when sleeping in wool compared to cotton sleepwear.[1]

I point this out not because I encourage you to switch sleepwear, since most sleep experts agree that whatever you feel most comfortable in will typically serve you best. But I want you to make sure that what you wear is meeting that need. If it's not, just consider what sleep attire may be the coziest and which may be shutting off your shut-eye.

Exercise

On this day, you'll continue to walk side by side with God. But instead of spending only fifty minutes, you'll walk with Him for sixty minutes. This amount of time is indeed a commitment, and as on previous days, if you need to divide up that time into several smaller Walks, that's understandable. But if possible, allow yourself that hour with Him to recognize how blessed you are to be able to have this time with Him.

It's so easy to look at having to spend even more time exercising as a burden instead of the blessing it really is. On this day, you're allowing yourself ten minutes more with Him than you had the day before, and that is something to be celebrated, for every minute spent alone with Him is another opportunity to draw closer to Him.

Nutrition

In the Genesis passage cited above, we are told how to nourish our bodies, and the things God created as food for us have not changed throughout time. What is available today is exactly what He created for us at the creation of the world and continues to provide for us now. So today and every day throughout Seven Sundays, look at the ingredients of everything you eat.

As you read each food label, don't concentrate on calories, grams of fat, or other numbers that most people typically home in on. Instead, look at each ingredient and ask: Am I seeing what He has provided for me? Is this one of the things God created for me to eat? Or is this ingredient man-made?

- If the answer is that the ingredient is man-made, odds are it's not something your body will be able to utilize and benefit from.
- If the answer is yes, that God provided the ingredient, odds are it has everything your body needs, so long as it's eaten in moderation.

The truth is, you don't need a background in nutrition to know the difference between what is healthy and what is not. Most times, the words we aren't quite clear on (or just have a hard time pronouncing) are typically additives and chemicals placed in our foods to serve as a sweetener or salt, a texture-changer, an artificial flavor or coloring, a taste-enhancing fat, or a preservative. They are ingredients that aren't placed there to make the foods you're eating healthier. Instead they are included to either get you to consume more of those foods or to make them more convenient to prepare and/or eat.

Once you separate what He has given us from what He has not, you start noticing the obvious difference between healthy and unhealthy foods. What is good for us has always been good for us— the foods that God provides: things like fruits and vegetables, whole grains, lean meats and fish, and other food sources that have existed since biblical times. Much of what is bad for us are the foods that didn't exist until recently—foods created by man, either out of a desire to provide convenience or to encourage temptation.

Unhealthy foods were never part of God's plan, and yet they exist. Is it any wonder that we struggle with our weight or our health in relation to our diets? Simply put, we're not listening to His initial instructions on what we were always meant to consume. That's why it's so important to bring yourself back to today's honoring thought whenever you question what to eat. It reminds us that God is the creator of all things and that maintaining better dietary habits isn't about being healthier and fit. It's about staying true to His plans for us.

DAY 7 (SATURDAY)

Concede

Father, I surrender to the fact that there is nothing I can do to receive more of Your grace other than believe in You. I realize that I can't do this day without Your grace. Reveal to me the areas in my life where there might be unbelief, so that I might receive more of Your unmerited favor on this day. Thank You, Father. Amen.

Honor

Some people believe that in order to receive God's grace, we must perform specific actions. But God's grace is unmerited, and even though we don't deserve His grace, He gives it to us anyway. Know on this day that it's through your belief in God that you always travel straight toward Him. Ephesians 2:8–9 illustrates that point:

> For it is by grace that you have been saved through faith. And this is not of yourselves, but it is the gift of God; not as a result of works, so that no one will boast or take credit in any way.

This is the relationship I want you to understand as you continue on this journey. Even though you're performing specific tasks, it's not through these works that you receive His grace. Never think that you have failed if you miss a workout, mess up on your diet, or find it impossible to complete certain offerings. His love and grace are already present for you. You're already saved through faith alone.

Offer

Reaching out to someone who is sick and visiting with them symbolizes grace. To make such an offering has an impact that's hard to define. Your very presence is a more powerful gesture to someone who is ailing than you might recognize. By making someone smile, your visit could just help them heal.

Unfortunately, we all know someone who isn't doing well. So today spend some time with them. This day is about being intentionally aware that there are others out there who could certainly use a warm smile and an earnest visit. Today is also about getting you to appreciate what you have in regards to your current health. Sometimes we don't count our blessings as often as we should, but by making an effort on this day, this offering will also help you appreciate your well-being.

Ideally, I would prefer this offering to take place today, but if connecting is impossible due to scheduling, a conflict with visiting hours, or not being able to reach someone, then at least get the ball in motion today to arrange a visit to someone somewhere along your Seven Sundays journey. Just the process of putting something on your calendar is a pledge to take that step.

Sleep

Today observe the brightness and volume of your environment several hours before you usually fall asleep.

- Is the house or apartment well-lit—and does it need to be?
- Are you sitting close to a light source?
- How loud is your space?
- Are there multiple sounds coming from different directions (two or more TVs, tablets, phones, for example)?

The more distractions that surround us prior to sleep, the more information our bodies are taking in, whether we are conscious of it or not. Those distractions can make it harder for us to turn off our brains and bring our spirit to rest when it's time for bed. Right now, you'll change nothing. All I ask is that you remain aware of what might be stimulating both your body and your spirit at a time when it should begin to subtly slow down.

Exercise

Today is an Acknowledge-Pray-Rest Day. Allow your body to recover from what you accomplished with your Worship Walks on Days 5 and 6. If you wish to walk with God on this day, you may do so as long as your Worship Walk doesn't exceed thirty minutes and you maintain a relaxed, comfortable pace. Also, if you wish to be active on this day, that is fine as well. Whatever activity you choose should be something that doesn't overexert you, so that your body is prepared for the week to come.

Nutrition

The people around us can have both a conscious and an unconscious effect on our actions. Today, on a day that we typically find ourselves eating with others at some point, carefully look at the foods you choose and focus on the following:

- Do the eating habits of those you're dining with mimic yours—or do your eating habits mimic theirs?
- Did you feel compelled to eat something so as not to offend someone?
- Did you rush to make a food choice because you felt pressured to order quickly?

Recognizing that what we eat is sometimes dictated by those around us, we learn that we're not as in control of what we put in our bodies as we should be. But if we find that others follow our lead, it's a reminder that we hold some responsibility when it comes to someone else's body as well.

From this day forth, take ownership of what you eat. More important, ask yourself if your eating habits are those you would wish to pass on to someone you love. Sometimes by merely having these thoughts in mind, you'll find that your specific dietary decisions may positively change.

DAY 8 (SUNDAY)

THE SECOND SUNDAY

The Week of Elevation
(Days 8 through 14)

You've managed to accomplish so much of God's work in a short period through the offerings of the previous week. You've also begun to devote more time to Him through your Worship Walks, and you've approached certain aspects of your life with an honest eye, knowing that He loves you and is always there for you, no matter what.

Through this handful of offerings, not only should you begin to feel your spirit growing stronger, but you should also start seeing their effects on others, whether through a smile or a stronger bond. Soon you'll begin to notice your physical body growing stronger. Before you begin, take this moment to go through each offering from last week to remind yourself how you felt after accomplishing each one:

- If you were nervous at first, remember how your apprehensions were soothed during and afterward as a result of the good you were doing.
- If certain offerings surprised you, think about why. Was it because of how good it felt to perform them or because of how much of a difference they seemed to make in someone else's life? Think about how easy it could be to re-create that feeling once again through the same considerate actions.
- If you think you could have tried harder, cast away any guilt and be proud of yourself instead—and give yourself credit for the effort you put in.
- If you couldn't complete specific offerings, think forward and try to figure out where those neglected offerings may find a home in your schedule next week.
- Finally, if you haven't performed a particular offering, would you have ever connected with the person or individuals you positively affected, or even met them in the first place? Let your actions of yesterday remind you of the new connections and stronger relationships you now have acquired in the space of just one week.

During this next week, you will lift yourself up by incorporating certain things into your life that accomplish exactly that. Over the next seven days, you'll add specific foods, exercise routines, and other elements that lift both the spiritual body and the physical body. You'll also be performing offerings that will raise up others in various ways as well. But today just let yourself rest, restore, and reflect.

Concede

Thank you, Father, for this day. It's the opportunity to strengthen my spirit and body. I choose to worship You regardless of how I may feel.

I ask that Your presence come in and break any obstacles that may be holding me back from victory today. I'm here to worship You in spirit and truth. Thank You, Father, Amen.

Honor

On this second Sunday, my hope is that you'll be immersed in other passages of the Bible as you worship. But bring one specific verse— Psalm 104:1—to the forefront:

> *Bless and affectionately praise the Lord, O my soul!*
> *O Lord my God, You are very great;*
> *You are clothed with splendor and majesty.*

This scripture's entire focus is elevating Him with praise, something we should be doing every day in His name. But as you read this passage throughout the day, remind yourself that every action and every step set in place over the next seven days is meant to uplift you, just as these words are intended to elevate Him.

Offer

Even though each Sunday along this journey is a day for rest and recovery, you will always perform an offering of some kind. Today that offering will be in the form of displaying some sort of encouragement on social media.

Facebook, Twitter, Instagram, and other forms of social media can often be used to shame, insult, or disparage. Even when they're being used positively, they can also be leaned upon in a way that disconnects us from others. They can make it easy to "like" something or give it a "thumbs-up," instead of choosing more intimate opportunities to connect.

On this day, instead of posting on your own social media pages about yourself, look online for others who have shared something personal—an act that shows they've done something honorable that truly makes the world a better place. Then go beyond the cursory response and craft a short paragraph that's thoughtful and upbeat—one that encourages and shows that you're genuinely proud and happy about their successes or well-being. Better still, use their post as an ice-breaking opportunity to reach out and praise their actions, either in person or over the phone. Whichever way you decide to connect, your only thought should be to make that person know how proud you are of them today.

Sleep

Last week, you became more aware of a few potential issues that could be affecting your sleep. But even though you weren't asked to change much along the way, this next week will be different.

Over the next seven days, you'll begin to make subtle additions to your sleep environment to create a more peaceful, healthy place to rest your head. The only thing to consider in preparation for this week will be to purchase an essential oil (one known to promote sleep) that you will use on Day 9. If you don't already have one at hand, turn to the "Sleep" section of Day 9 to see what options you have to choose from.

Exercise

During this next week, you'll switch from merely walking with Him to also working out with Him. Over the next seven days, you'll begin adding strength-training exercises to your workout; you'll be asked to perform certain exercises using dumbbells indoors, in addition to specific bodyweight exercises outdoors after your Worship

Walk. But today just reflect on a few things to prepare for the days ahead:

- Did you finish your Worship Walks last week at a location where you feel you can perform bodyweight exercises safely? You should end up at a place that is both flat and stable.
- Will you be comfortable exercising at that location? If not, then think about an area where you can walk and not feel self-conscious exercising afterward.
- Do you have a pair of dumbbells and either a sturdy chair or bench? If not, ask a friend if you can borrow these pieces of equipment so you're all ready to go for this coming Friday (when you'll perform the exercises for the first time).

This week, you'll also be asked to hike, bike, or swim on Tuesday, so if you need to arrange anything to make that possible, today is an ideal day to initiate that step. However, know that if you can't get access to equipment (or if this option isn't convenient for you), you'll be presented with an alternative that requires nothing more than a pair of shoes.

Nutrition

You've now become more aware of your nutritional habits, along with what is present in many of the foods you typically turn to for nourishment. You've also spent some time thinking about what you're striving for when it comes to your diet.

This week may be the first time you have ever come face-to-face with your diet in a pure, honest way because you've performed this task with God by your side instead of alone. If so, then take pride in that honesty because it's only when we're honest with ourselves that we can ever truly change.

Also, know this: We are all creatures of habit, especially when it comes to our diet. What we eat in a given week is, for all intents and purposes, what we typically eat every week. That doesn't mean I want you to stop keeping a food journal. In fact, I urge that you continue the process throughout Seven Sundays to see how much your dietary habits have changed along the way.

To prepare for the next seven days, I also encourage you to look ahead at the nutrition portions of Days 9 through 14. That's because each day, you'll be introducing at least one or two of the following Faith-Full Foods into your diet:

Healthy fats
Healthy whole grains
Protein-rich foods
Nutrient-dense fruits
Oatmeal (and other high-fiber foods)
Vegetables
Green tea
All-natural sweetening foods
Enzyme-rich foods
Sea salt (and other all-natural herbs and spices)

Collectively, the ten Faith-Full Foods—each a nourishing, nutrient-rich, all-natural food source—are the types of foods you should be seeking every time you have a meal or snack throughout your Seven Sundays journey. These all-natural foods stand as a testament to the fact that God indeed has provided everything we need nutritionally— that the foods that genuinely serve us best are the same ones that He has blessed us with, and not those created by man.

Finally, know this: although I expect you to taste each of the Faith-Full Foods this week—and I'll offer instruction on how many servings would be ideal—you're only encouraged to "do your best" to incorporate them into your diet on a daily basis from that point forward. This journey—first and foremost—is about enriching your relationship with Him, and part of that comes from consuming only foods that He has provided us. How far you cultivate that connection is entirely up to you along your journey. All I ask is that you try.

DAY 9 (MONDAY)

Concede

Father, I surrender all the heaviness over to You. I declare Your abundance of favor, love, and grace in my life today. I will experience a new rhythm in my life that I've never experienced before. Today things will work for me and not against me. I will see You turn around all things for my good so that You can be glorified. Thank You, Father. Amen.

Honor

Start your day with the verse Psalm 23:5, and think about it throughout your day:

> *You prepare a table before me in the presence of my enemies.*
> *You have anointed and refreshed my head with oil;*
> *My cup overflows.*

The act of anointing—the placing of oil on a person as a token of honor, as a means of healing or comfort, or as a symbol of dedication—is present throughout the Bible. And in many cases, the oil itself is often viewed as a token of the Holy Spirit, as seen in examples such as 1 John 2:20: *But you have an anointing from the Holy One, and all of you know.*

Through anointing, things begin to flow in your life.

A lot of times, we feel that we are somehow trapped in one place, and we feel anxious, sad, or defeated. But what you need to remember is that the Holy Spirit continually flows through you, even in times when you think that your life is in a rut. You are perpetually being anointed by the Holy Spirit, and when you walk with Jesus (the Anointed One), His love flows through you as well. Today (and every day moving forward) remind yourself that in moments when you are still, you are *always* moving forward.

Offer

Today show your affection for someone you love by spending at least fifteen minutes giving them a massage (shoulders, feet, or full-body).

A deep sense of affection and connection is expressed through physical touch. And just fifteen minutes of massage has been proven to both increase oxytocin (a hormone known to aid social bonding) and reduce adrenocorticotropin, the hormone responsible for stimulating the adrenals to release cortisol.[1] Having elevated amounts of cortisol in your body can lead to hypertension, a suppressed immune system, and weight gain (among other negative effects), so your offering isn't just making someone feel more relaxed; it's helping them heal from within.

If you don't feel comfortable performing a massage, you could always buy one for somebody. Offering something you could have easily have given yourself is a kind gesture that also shows selflessness. As this other person releases stress, they are left with little choice but to think about how they came to be in that relaxing position in the first place—through a genuine act of benevolence.

But know that there are other ways to express the connection you have with someone on this day. It can be as simple as an unexpected hug, a hand on a shoulder, or shaking someone's hand with a little more enthusiasm (wrapping your other hand around theirs, smiling, and making eye contact to show how happy you are to see them).

Sleep

The scent of certain therapeutic oils, either applied or diffused before bedtime, can sometimes help induce sleep by easing stress and placing your body in a more restful state. Tonight try experimenting with an essential oil known to promote sleep. The best scents to explore on this night—and every night from this day forward—can include:

Roman chamomile

Lavender

Neroli

Valerian

Frankincense

Ylang ylang

Jasmine

Cedarwood

If you don't want to invest in a diffuser, that's entirely fine. Instead place ten to twenty drops of any pharmaceutical or therapeutic grade essential oil into a small spray bottle, add three to four ounces of water, shake, then spray the mixture lightly on your pillow, or gently apply a drop or two of the mix on your wrists, the back of your neck, and behind your ears. You can find pharmaceutical or therapeutic-grade essential oils online through Amazon, at most health food stores, and at most drugstores.

Exercise

Today you'll walk outside with Him for forty-five minutes, then do a mini-circuit using two outdoor exercises—the Push-up and the Lunge. These two exercises, when combined, offer the perfect, bare-bones full-body workout. The Push-up strengthens the muscles throughout your chest, shoulders, and triceps while also engaging your core muscles. The Lunge works your legs and glutes, as well as your core muscles, which need to be engaged to help you remain balanced.

Immediately after your Worship Walk, you'll move through both exercises back-to-back with no rest in between.

- Start by performing Push-ups for ten repetitions.
- Next, you'll perform Lunges for ten repetitions (each leg).
- That's one circuit! Rest for one minute by walking (or standing) in place, then repeat the mini-circuit once more for a total of two circuits.

If performing these exercises outside makes you feel self-conscious, just recognize that you've just spent forty-five minutes walking and talking with God, so you should be filled with a sense of peace and love that leaves you feeling less insecure. But at times when that's not enough, think about several things as you exercise outdoors.

First, express gratitude for the opportunity to exercise outdoors surrounded by many of the things that He's created for you, and try to feel grateful that you have a body able to perform these movements. And remind yourself that if others are watching, you may be inspiring them to do something similar for themselves.

We've all watched others being active outdoors. During those moments, what did you feel toward that person? Was it ever the things you're afraid others may be expressing toward you—like laughter or disrespect? Or did they merely remind you about your own activity level? Odds are, you were left either motivated or unaffected, which is exactly what others are feeling when they see you exercise outdoors. My hope is that you'll inspire instead of simply being ignored, and that should be your hope as well.

If you find yourself feeling awkward or embarrassed performing the strength-training portion today, try reaching deep down into yourself and overcoming that feeling of nervousness. Remind yourself that every set of eyes on you isn't judgmental. Most people will see you for what you are in that moment: an inspiration. You'll be surprised how that one simple thought will remove your fear and replace it with faith.

Nutrition

Today you'll begin to incorporate not one but two types of Faith-Full Foods into your routine: healthy fats and healthy whole grains.

Healthy Fats

When weight loss is a goal, many people make the mistake of turning their back on all forms of fat. But not all forms of fat are created equal.

Unsaturated fats (the kind that remain liquid at room temperature) are divided into two types: monounsaturated fats and polyunsaturated fats. Both are healthy in moderation, helping to not only lower harmful LDL cholesterol and stabilize your blood sugar, but also curb appetite, reduce inflammation, lower your blood pressure, and provide your body with fat-soluble vitamins, such as A, D, E, and K.

That's why I'd like you to try eating foods containing healthy fats from unsaturated sources more often, including cold-water fish (such as mackerel, salmon, and tuna), avocados, plant oils (canola, flaxseed, walnut, peanut, sunflower, sesame, soybean, and olive oil), nuts and seeds, and all-natural peanut butter. If possible, strive for four servings of healthy fats a day. It's not difficult. Three ounces of fatty fish, a half ounce of seeds or nuts, a quarter of an avocado, or a tablespoon of all-natural peanut butter are all perfect serving sizes.

Healthy Whole Grains

There's a big difference when it comes to whole-grains—grains that remain unprocessed and intact, as God intended them to be—and refined grains (processed grains that are treated to remove one or more of these three essential pieces: bran, germ, or endosperm). The process is meant to make a grain last longer, but it's not a move that will help you live a healthier life.

For example, I *love* Ezekiel bread, which is made from sprouted organic whole grains that are packed with fiber and nutrients, including iron and magnesium. Bread (and other products) made from refined grains, on the other hand, are starchier, are typically stripped of their nutrients and fiber, and tend to be loaded with a variety of man-made chemicals.

Even worse, products made from refined grains also spike your blood sugar, triggering the release of insulin, a hormone that stabilizes blood-sugar levels. How does it do that? By storing all that sugar rushing through the body mostly (and unfortunately) as unwanted body fat. On the other hand, whole grains (or foods made from whole grains) take longer to digest, which slows down the absorption of sugar into the bloodstream and prevents your body from experiencing an insulin rush that can cause you to store fat.

Try to seek out more whole-grain foods, such as quinoa, wild or brown rice, bulgur, couscous, and oats. If possible, strive for three to five servings a day, which is possible if you make sure that every meal and snack contains a serving of some form of whole-grain food. But if you're uncertain about any whole-grain product, just look at the label.

According to the American Heart Association, you should choose one that contains at least one of the following as the product's "very first" ingredient:[2]

Whole wheat

Graham flour

Oatmeal

Whole oats

Brown rice

Wild rice

Whole-grain corn

Popcorn

Whole-grain barley

Whole-wheat bulgur

Whole rye

DAY 10 (TUESDAY)

Concede

Father, I've been held in bondage, but on this day, I am no longer a slave to fear. On this day, I and everyone else around me will experience the fullness of my heart. I will love fearlessly like a child and pursue everything that is good in my life with all the passion within me. And I will hold nothing back. Thank You, Father. Amen.

Honor

One of my favorite verses is 1 Samuel 13:14.

> *"But now your kingdom shall not endure. The Lord has sought out for Himself a man after His own heart, and the Lord has appointed him as leader and ruler over His people, because you have not kept what the Lord commanded you."*

There are very few places in the Bible where it speaks about anyone being a person after His own heart. But in these verses, this is what is said of David. The compliment to David is magnanimous, but what it also reveals to us is that God sees inside our hearts.

It means that who we are inside is far more important than where others may rank us in society or the various forms of measurement that others sometimes judge us by. In other words, He is not judging us by our appearance, possessions, or occupations. He is looking at our hearts—always—to see where they measure up against His. On this day, remind yourself that He always sees inside yours. Make Him proud of what He finds.

Offer

Today you will support someone financially. The size of the support doesn't matter. What is important is that it's done anonymously.

Giving should never be transactional—meaning we should never expect something in return. It should always be about doing something merely because it's the right thing to do. On this day, I hope you will give, knowing there won't be a thank-you, a pat on the back, or a receipt for tax purposes. It's about giving as much as you can without expecting to get anything in return—most important, recognition for your effort.

The person receiving the gift sees not only benevolence, but the fact that there was someone of character behind it. So you will be offering financial support, but, more important, you'll offer proof that people with good hearts are out there. Maybe it will inspire the recipient to act in the same anonymously charitable way someday.

When you give anonymously, that act is also solely between you and God. It's a secret the two of you share, and I believe that God rewards generosity as well as humility. He takes pride in those who give without need of recognition. Whatever you give this day, don't share any details with friends, family, or anyone else you may come in contact with. This should be between you and Him.

It doesn't have to be much, especially if you don't have the funds to give. But if you're not sure who to give to, being aware of others' needs is the first place to start. Look around at others in your life and listen to what they seem to be lacking. For some, it may be a financial need, while for others, it might be something physical, such as clothing, books, or toys. If you hear about a problem you could solve, try to fulfill the need in a way that allows you to be anonymous.

It could be as simple as putting a gift card in an envelope, writing nothing on it except the phrase "Thank you for being you." Or you could place two tickets to a movie, passes to a theme park or museum, or general admission to something that someone may not have the financial means to visit or see. Just listen, and then let the Spirit work through you to provide an answer that allows you to be unidentified.

Sleep

If you're in the habit of washing your face before bedtime, avoid splashing cold water on your face to close your pores afterward. This can bring your body into a more alert state that could make it more difficult to ease into sleep. Instead stick with warm water from this point forward, or try washing your face at least thirty minutes before bedtime if you need to close your pores with cold water.

Exercise

On this day, hike, bike, or swim—whichever activity you're most comfortable with—for thirty minutes total. Ideally, I would prefer you to be outside, but if that's not possible today, it's fine to use a stationary bike, treadmill, or indoor pool.

If none of these options are possible, convenient, or appealing to you, then you can perform a walk/jog workout instead. To do it, you'll walk for thirty minutes, but instead of walking at a normal pace, just walk at an easy pace for one to two minutes, then jog for fifteen to thirty seconds. Continue to alternate between walking and jogging for the duration of the workout (thirty minutes total).

There are several reasons I prefer that you try one of these three activities. First, there's something to be said about adding a new stimulus and placing yourself in a new environment. It adds a little pep to your step by keeping things fresh and forcing you to get even further out of your comfort zone. It also shakes things up for your body. Because every activity incorporates a different series of muscles, the more you mix up your routine, the more you'll challenge the body in different ways, allowing you to build a stronger, leaner body from head to toe.

Nutrition

Today you will try to incorporate not one, but two types of Faith-Full Foods into your routine: protein-rich foods, as well as nutrient-dense fruits.

Protein-rich Foods

While most people associate protein—the macronutrient found commonly in eggs, milk, fish, and meats—as being essential for building and maintaining lean muscle, what's not as well known is that our bodies use protein to make, grow, and repair many things within us, including bone, cartilage, meniscus, ligaments, and tendons. In fact, protein is the building block behind every cell within you. That's right—every single cell.

The only problem is that protein is also the only one among the three macronutrients (fat and carbohydrates rounding out the trio) that your body can't store. That's why, ideally, I would like you to have one serving of lean protein as part of every meal or snack.

How Much—and What—to Eat

A typical serving of protein can come in many forms. Adding any of the following suggestions works perfectly, depending on your tastes:

Three to four ounces of seafood, poultry, lean beef, or game meat

A handful of nuts

A six- to eight-ounce serving of dairy (milk, cottage cheese, or yogurt)

One or two eggs

However, if you're a vegetarian, know that He has provided us with other high-protein foods, such as black beans (or beans of any kind), tofu, and edamame.

Nutrient-dense Fruits

Loaded with vitamins (such as vitamins A and C) and minerals (like potassium and folate), most fruits are also water-rich and full of fiber as well. The end result of all that goodness in one package? Eating them on a regular basis has been shown to reduce your risk of many chronic diseases and health issues, including heart disease and stroke, certain cancers, bone loss, and type 2 diabetes, just to name a few.

If you're concerned that eating too much fruit might raise your blood sugar to dangerous levels, let me ease your fears. Although fruit contains naturally occurring sugars that do have an effect on your blood sugar, it also contains a lot of nutrients that help your body stay strong and healthy. Plus, when was the last time you couldn't stop eating fruit? Exactly. That's because the fiber and water they contain fill you up so you're not as likely to eat more than you should (unlike foods that contain added sugars, which tend to have fewer nutrients, water, and fiber, as well as more calories).

How Much—and What—to Eat

You goal should be to reach for a minimum of two cups (for women) and three cups (for men) of fruit per day. If you're not sure what to eat, try eating the rainbow. The color of fruits is in most cases an indicator of the nutrients they contain. In that respect, God has made it easy to keep our bodies balanced nutritionally. By simply eating a wide variety of colors each week, you'll be taking in a wider range of nutrients.

That said, a few among God's bounty that stand out (even though I encourage eating any type of fruit) include:

Bananas: A great source of both fiber and potassium, a nutrient that prevents muscle cramps, they help regulate blood pressure and stimulate the formation of red blood cells.

Pears: Eaten with the skin, an average-size pear contains five grams of soluble fiber that can significantly reduce blood cholesterol levels and lower your risk of heart disease.[1]

Blackberries, raspberries, blueberries, and cherries: Fiber-rich, their phytonutrients and antioxidants (particularly anthocyanin) may also help reverse the memory loss associated with aging[2] and reduce inflammation.[3]

Papayas: Fortified with vitamins (including A, C, and E), they also contain lycopene, which may reduce your risk of cancer.[4]

Plums and apricots: Packed with vitamins A and C, they also have a fair number of anthocyanins and potassium.

Citrus fruits: Every kind contains vitamin C, fiber, and flavonoids that defend against heart-related diseases.[5]

Cranberries: Eaten fresh, they have been proven to increase your HDL (the good cholesterol).[6]

DAY 11 (WEDNESDAY)

Concede

Father, Your Word says that if I cast all my worries and anxieties over to You, I will experience a wave of peace that transcends all understanding. I want to experience the quiet and rest that comes from Your peace. I surrender my life to You—so that I can become one with You. Thank You, Father. Amen.

Honor

On Day 4, you worked toward overcoming fear, but that doesn't mean doubt will never find its way back into your life along this journey, particularly during this second week. With the introduction of so many new things this week, you might feel overwhelmed. That's why, at this midpoint in the week, it's worthwhile to think about Philippians 4:6–7.

Do not be anxious or worried about anything, but in everything by prayer and petition with thanksgiving, continue to make your requests known to God. And the peace of God, which transcends all understanding, stands guard over your hearts and your minds in Christ Jesus.

The truth is, it's natural for specific worries and anxieties to find their way into our lives. But it's our worries and concerns that make us break away from being at one with God. They make us unsettled and remove us from a place of peace.

Philippians 4:6–7 is a reminder that you can cast your worries, anxieties, and fears to God. And once you do that, you become connected with Him and are left to feel a solidarity and sense of harmony that removes all doubt. So if you doubt this day—and at any moment along the journey—know that no matter what your circumstances are, no matter what you're dealing with at this very moment, it is possible to be at peace right now.

Offer

Everyone has a skill, talent, or some knowledge they can share. Everyone also has the ability to teach, no matter how shy or unqualified you may believe yourself to be. That's why on this day you will seek out someone—or a group of people—to teach without compensation.

When you share your skills and talents, it's not just an opportunity to improve someone else's life. It can also help reignite the passion you have for what you do and what you're good at. Seeing the impact your skill or talent has through another person's eyes can be a reminder of the gifts God has blessed you with—of what makes you truly special.

Figuring out where to start can be the hardest step. You may have many skills and talents to choose from, or you may believe that you have none. First, assess yourself. If nothing comes to mind, it may be that you're not giving yourself enough credit for what you know how to do.

I find it's quite common for many humble Christians to be modest about their own self-worth and what makes them unique. If this is you, then try turning to friends and family members who know you best, tell them your day's assignment, and ask them to think of a few things they believe you could teach or share with others.

Sleep

The sense of peace that God brings us washes over all worry, but we can also bring on a sense of peace when we slow our breathing. Becoming conscious of our breath allows us to connect with Him, as well as with our bodies. That's why as you lie in bed tonight—and every night moving forward—just breathe through your nose as deeply and as slowly as possible, allowing your belly and not your chest to rise, for a minimum of fifteen to twenty breaths.

When you breathe only through your chest, you mainly utilize the upper third of the lungs, which means they take in less air and deliver less oxygen to your bloodstream. But when you take deeper, fuller, slower breaths, you not only receive more oxygen-rich air; this kind of breathing also triggers a parasympathetic response that promotes relaxation.

Even though this technique is ideal for inducing sleep, it's not something you need to reserve only for the end of each day. In fact, the more often you use this technique throughout the day, the more your body and spirit will be at peace.

Find times during the day to take a minute or two to slow down your breath. It could be every time you walk into a store, before answering any e-mails or texts, or right before engaging someone in conversation. No matter when you implement it, you'll discover that you'll approach that situation with a calmer perspective and have more clarity at that moment.

Exercise

Today is an Acknowledge-Pray-Rest Day. Allow your body to recover from what you accomplished on Days 9 and 10. However, if you wish to walk with God on this day, you may do so as long as your Worship Walk doesn't exceed thirty minutes and you maintain an easy, comfortable pace. If you wish to spend additional time with Him, I encourage you to spend that time in prayer to allow your body to recover and heal.

Nutrition

Today you'll be incorporating a Faith-Full Food that both cleanses your body and helps move things along.

Oatmeal (and Other High-fiber Foods)

Fiber-rich foods promote digestive health, control blood-sugar levels, help prevent type 2 diabetes, and reduce your risk of heart disease by lowering cholesterol by as much as 15 percent, among other things. They also keep you feeling fuller longer, which can keep you from consuming more food than your body needs during the day.

Basically, if you're eating enough of them, they help maintain a sense of order, balance, and peace throughout your body all day long. Our bodies require twenty-five to thirty grams of fiber daily, but most of us never see half that amount in our diets. That's why at every meal or snack, you should try to be conscious of the fiber you're eating.

By eating more whole grains and fruits, you'll most likely be getting some fiber. And when you begin to add another Faith-Full Food on Day 12 (vegetables), you will begin to enjoy more. And there are other ways you can add even more of this vital Faith-Full Food into your day:

- Try sprinkling any of these fiber-packed add-ons onto your meals: ground flaxseed, beans, sesame seeds, carrot shavings, wheat germ, oat bran, and cocoa powder.

- Mix any of the following into your foods: berries, chopped onions, canned pumpkin, low-sodium sauerkraut, and sliced avocado.
- Opt for almond or peanut butter over regular butter (both have one gram of fiber per tablespoon, while butter has zero).

DAY 12 (THURSDAY)

Concede

Father, I am hungry to elevate my physical and spiritual body today. I realize that this will be no easy task, but Your Word says that we can do all things through Christ, Who strengthens us. Therefore, I surrender to You so that I can harness this amazing power that comes from Your Holy Spirit. I believe that new levels will be reached on this day. Thank You, Father. Amen.

Honor

On this day, ponder how the Word of God works within each of us as a seed. One of my beloved set of verses that exemplifies what to contemplate throughout the day is Genesis 2:7–9:

> *Then the Lord God formed man from the dust of the ground, and breathed into his nostrils the breath of life; and the man became a living being. And the Lord God planted a garden (oasis) in the east, in Eden; and He put the man whom He had formed (created) there. And the Lord God caused to grow from the ground every tree that is desirable and pleasing to the sight and good (suitable, pleasant) for food; the tree of life was also in the midst*

*of the garden, and the tree of the knowledge (recognition) of good
and evil.*

These verses—the knowledge that immediately after our Creation,
the Garden of Eden was planted and we were placed there—illustrate
the importance God places on what is grown from the earth. Every
tree, plant, and form of vegetation was created by Him, which is why
it's so important not only to appreciate everything you see that's growing around you but to take part in enjoying as many of these blessings, given to us throughout the day, as possible.

Offer

You'll serve Him today by planting words of encouragement into
those whom you come in contact with. Those seeds of encouragement could come in the form of speaking scripture, telling someone you love them and believe in them, or simply speaking the
truth. All of these are equally important seeds when we converse
with people.

Just don't be concerned with whether or not every seed will take
root. You may not see their bounty for a long time or ever be privy to
the impact your words have on that person's life. Or you may instantly
see the effect of particular seeds you plant along the way.

Don't worry about how many seeds you plant, but merely make an
effort to continuously plant them at every opportunity from the time
you wake up until the time you go to sleep. Also, don't count how
many people you've made smile or left fulfilled. Instead just count on
the fact that what you're doing is making an impact, both on others
and on yourself.

And make sure you're not reserving these words of encouragement
just for people you know. I encourage you to make a point of planting the seeds in people whom you may see every day but do not pay

attention to. It might be the person you buy coffee from, a coworker you never had the pleasure to meet, or perhaps even a perfect stranger.

Sleep

For a seed to reach its maximum potential, it not only needs the right amount of water and sunlight, but it also needs to stay at the perfect temperature. If the environment is too cold or too warm, it doesn't matter how much you water it or how much sunlight shines down.

The same applies to sleep. Before you climb into bed, you have to consider the "climate" around you. That's why today I encourage you to begin experimenting with the temperature of your bedroom. What few people realize is that your body temperature decreases to initiate sleep. Our bodies are designed to lower their internal temperature while we rest. That's how He hardwired us, which is why lowering the temperature of your bedroom can assist you with getting a deeper, more restorative night's sleep.

Tonight set the temperature in your bedroom to between 60 and 67 degrees. Your bedroom should feel cool, not warm and cozy. If lowering the temperature is impossible, you can try a variety of other things to cool your physical body down, such as keeping your feet out from under the covers, buying a cooling pillow, or even placing a small pillow in the freezer, then sticking it between your knees right before bedtime.

Exercise

Today you'll walk outside with Him for forty minutes, then do a mini-circuit of the remaining three outdoor exercises—the Moving Plank, the Burpee, and the Superman.

Immediately after your Worship Walk, you'll move through all three exercises back-to-back-to-back with no rest in between.

- Start by performing the Moving Plank for thirty seconds.
- From there, you'll perform Burpees for twelve repetitions.
- Finally, get on the ground, and do one set of Supermans for twenty repetitions.
- That's one circuit! Rest for one minute by walking (or standing) in place, then repeat the mini-circuit once more for a total of two circuits.

Nutrition

Just as you'll be concentrating on planting the Word of God—in yourself and in others—you'll be adding two nourishing Faith-Full Foods into your diet to help it grow.

Vegetables

You already may know that fresh vegetables are a tremendous natural source of vitamins, minerals, antioxidants, and other nutrients. You may also understand that a diet rich in veggies has been shown to reduce the risk of heart disease and stroke, many forms of cancer, and a variety of other chronic diseases. But what's also important to remember is that most vegetables are also low-glycemic foods that are not only low in calories but typically packed with fiber that leaves you feeling fuller longer, so you're less likely to overeat or, worse, turn to a Faith-Less Food in response to a craving.

Because of all that fiber, vegetables also take more time to digest, so they release smaller amounts of any natural sugars they may contain at a much slower, more consistent rate. The end result: Your body gets a steadier stream of energy from the vegetables you eat. That way, your blood sugar doesn't rise suddenly, preventing insulin from being released that can turn all that sugar into excess body fat.

How Much—and What—to Eat

As long as you're eating vegetables in their natural form—meaning you haven't breaded and fried them, gotten them from a can, or mixed them into any creamy sauces—you're free to eat as many as you like. At the very least, strive to have a minimum of two cups (for women) or three cups (for men) per day. However, there are two things to consider to ensure you're making the most of how they were intended to be eaten:

Always Explore His Bounty. Every vegetable has its own unique mix of nutrients. For example, broccoli contains sulforaphane, a potent phytochemical that helps fight cancer[1] and osteoarthritis,[2] and zucchini is rich in both lutein and zeaxanthin,[3] two phytonutrients that promote healthy eyesight,[4] while peppers and cabbage provide abundant amounts of vitamin C, which plays a crucial in maintaining the health of the physical body's connective tissue. By not sticking with the same handful of tried-and-true vegetables—and exploring as many of the twenty thousand edible vegetables He has provided us—you will greatly enhance the nutrition you are giving your physical body.

When in doubt, a simple way to guarantee a mix of nutrients is to consume at least one type of vegetable daily of the following colors:

Red (such as red cabbage, red bell pepper, tomatoes, and beets)

Orange/yellow (carrots, bell peppers, sweet potatoes, pumpkin, and butternut squash, for example)

Green (including spinach, kale, broccoli, artichokes, asparagus, rapini, mustard greens, and zucchini)

Blue/purple (such as eggplant, purple cabbage, endive, and purple asparagus)

White (including cauliflower, onions, mushrooms, and garlic)

Eat Them as He Intended. Eating vegetables with their edible peels intact boosts your fiber intake, so whenever possible, keep the skin on. Also, the richer and brighter a vegetable is (whether it's bright green, orange, red, or yellow) the more nutritionally dense it's likely to be—so look for the clues nature offers. Finally, whenever possible, choose organic.

When you turn to non-organic vegetables, you are most likely eating a GMO (a genetically modified organism), a vegetable that's had its DNA engineered and changed by man to take on certain characteristics, such as resistance to certain bugs or herbicides. Organic vegetables often don't appear to be as perfect or as large as those treated with chemical fertilizers and pesticides, but they are grown as God intended. As such, they are free of any negative health issues, and typically contain more vitamins and minerals than non-organic versions.

Green Tea

Instead of reaching for coffee or other beverages, try green tea instead. Green tea not only delivers a natural, plant-based source of caffeine, but it's been shown to improve blood flow and lower cholesterol. It's also teeming with both catechins and polyphenols, two vital antioxidants that have a huge effect on protecting your body and maintaining good health.

The catechins in green tea are believed to fight cellular damage and may be responsible for boosting your body's ability to burn stored fat for energy. The polyphenols found in green tea are equally beneficial, helping to prevent heart disease, diabetes, and cancer, while they also reduce inflammation in the body and reduce the risk of age-related brain changes.

The best way to brew it:

- Steep loose tea (instead of using pre-packaged bags). Ground-up tea leaves tend to lose both flavor and some nutrients, while loose tea tends to be richer in catechin and polyphenols.
- Never use boiling water, which can destroy catechins. The best temperature is water at about 150–170 degrees.

DAY 13 (FRIDAY)

Concede

Father, I declare that my body and spirit will unite and become one today, strengthening me from the inside out. Father, I cannot do it with my own strength. I need a heavenly strength that far surpasses my own. This newfound power will take me to a greater level than ever before. Thank You, Father. Amen.

Honor

Today I ask that you think about one verse in particular, and that's 1 Timothy 4:8.

> *For physical training is of some value, but godliness is of value in every thing and in every way, since it holds promise for the present life and for the life to come.*

This verse truly embodies what you're trying to accomplish throughout the Seven Sundays program. It tells us that taking care of ourselves through physical training is what God wants of us and that it holds value. But it's also a reminder that your journey should never be only about strengthening and reshaping yourself. This entire journey is about not only changing your body but enlightening you as well, and reinforcing that we need to have both outer strength and inner strength simultaneously.

Offer

Sometimes our offerings—despite how generous they may be—may feel less important when they're relatively easy to perform. Believe me when I say that smiling or praying for someone else are important offerings. But there's something to be said about performing an offering that requires both our spirit and our body. That's why today I encourage you to strive to do something physical for someone, some form of task or job that allows you to lend a hand—and your muscles—to get the job done.

You could do someone else's chores, such as dusting, vacuuming, doing dishes, or handling laundry. You could try asking a neighbor or friend if there are any responsibilities they've put on hold because they required some assistance from another. Or ask the church if there are any errands you could complete for them, or connect with a local organization or non-profit that would appreciate having your assistance.

If nothing comes to mind, you could try this: Allow your church leader to present the opportunity to the congregation next Sunday, letting everyone know that you have some free time that day to help anyone in need. I can assure you, there's always someone in the middle of some project who would gladly welcome your help. More important, hearing that selfless act presented in this setting may motivate others to raise their hands as well to offer assistance to those you couldn't help that day. You never know what you may encourage in others through a single altruistic gesture.

Why is this such an important step? When we read about Jesus in the Word of God, there are many things that are evident about Him. Yet beyond His kindness and wisdom, one thing we see throughout the Bible is how He always took a very hands-on approach to helping others.

But there is another reason that I ask you to do this, and that's the way it reminds us how blessed we are to be able to physically assist others. Instead of being sore or tired after your task, rejoice that you're blessed with a healthy body capable of aiding someone in the way that you have. And know that at the end of Seven Sundays, you'll be less tired and stronger, which means you'll be able to assist someone more often and with more energy and strength, potentially making an even larger positive impact on the lives of others.

Finally, really embrace this offering, because there will be times when I ask you to exercise but you may want to quit or put less effort into your workouts. On those days, when you can't find it within yourself to give it your all, remember how good you felt when you physically helped someone else. Remembering the good you were able to accomplish today, you may be inspired to stay the course when it comes to exercise, knowing that each workout will lead to a stronger body that is capable of stepping in and helping others whenever necessary.

Sleep

On Day 7, I asked that you observe the lights around you. Today try lowering the lights two or three hours before bedtime.

Lowering the lights may feel effortless, but its effect on your body is much greater than you might recognize. After all, God created us to be diurnal by nature, so as the sun sets, our bodies naturally begin to prepare for the act of sleep. By keeping the lights bright and then turning every light off immediately before bedtime, we disrupt His design and the way our bodies were meant to gradually slow down for the evening. This simple, subtle change works with that process, assisting in calming your mind and spirit at a slow, steady pace that eases you toward sleep.

Exercise

Today you'll undertake your first indoor workout of the journey. Just as it's important to work on both inner and outer strength, it's equally important to challenge yourself with a mix of both indoor and outdoor exercises. Bringing things indoors can sometimes give you more focus because there's less distraction; more important, it gives you access to certain fitness tools (such as dumbbells and benches) that tax your muscles in different ways.

Today you'll move through a circuit of all five indoor exercises in order—the Double-Pump Shoulder Press, the Dip, the Squat & Hold, the Step Up, and Bicycles. To perform this mini-circuit, you'll do all five exercises back-to-back-to-back with no rest in between.

- Start by performing the Double-Pump Shoulder Press for ten repetitions.
- From there, you'll perform Dips for ten repetitions.
- Next, you'll do Squat & Holds for ten repetitions.
- After that, you'll do Step Ups for ten repetitions (each leg).
- Finally, you'll get on the ground and do Bicycles for fifteen repetitions.
- Rest for one minute by walking (or standing) in place, then repeat the mini-circuit once more for a total of two circuits.

So, where's the Worship Walk? First, because your offering today is physical, I don't want your body to be too stressed. And even though you'll be focusing solely on a five-move, strength-training circuit, you'll be elevating your heart rate and improving your aerobic capacity as you perform the routine. Doing all five exercises one after the other, with little to no rest, is a more intense form of exercise that not only helps build lean muscle tissue, but also improves your cardiovascular health at the same time.

Nutrition

Today you will add two new Faith-Full foods, both of which will help your overall health.

All-Natural Sweetening Foods

Often we satisfy our sweet tooth with processed sugar and artificial sweeteners, instead of turning to what God has already provided us. By adding certain naturally sweetened foods in moderation (no more than one to two teaspoons daily), you have the peace of mind that you're ingesting something created to naturally appease that desire, as opposed to something man-made that could be affecting your overall health over time. For the rest of this journey, when you need to use sugar in a recipe, in your coffee, or to sweeten something in a pinch, try turning to all-natural sources such as:

Raw honey

Coconut sugar

Blackstrap molasses

Date sugar

100 percent stevia extract (which is unprocessed)

All-natural maple syrup

Enzyme-rich Foods

Our bodies have a natural harmony with nature, and certain foods provide not only nutrients, but also components beyond nutrients that can assist us from the inside. Some foods contain enzymes or other healthy bacteria that help break down and assist the digestion of food. This not only allows more nutrients to be released from the healthy foods we're eating; it also gives our body a break so it doesn't have to work as hard at every meal. When we eat processed foods, many of the enzymes God has placed inside food for us are stripped away.

That's why, starting today, I want to encourage you to try incorporating enzyme-rich foods into your diet as often as possible. Some of my favorite options include:

Apricots (teeming with enzymes, they're also rich in invertase, a helpful enzyme that converts sucrose into energy)

Avocados (full of healthy fats, but also the enzyme lipase, which helps break down fat)

Bananas (packed with potassium, as well as amylase and maltase, two enzymes that help break down carbohydrates and malt sugar)

Kimchi, kombucha, Greek yogurt, or any form of fermented vegetable (all are rich in helpful bacteria—probiotics—that may boost the immune system and positively affect digestive health)

Pineapples (which contain bromelain, a natural anti-inflammatory)

Each offers its own set of nutritional benefits, so try not to stick with just one. The more you explore them, the better off your body will be.

DAY 14 (SATURDAY)

Concede

Father, I feel like I have lost my substance. I ask that You help enhance and add meaning to my life again. Help me regain my flavor so I can add balance and hope to whatever and to whomever You call me to. I'm here to be a good steward and to preserve what is good for You. Thank You, Father. Amen.

Honor

Today Matthew 5:13 will be your source of inspiration:

> *"You are the salt of the earth; but if the salt has lost its taste, how can it be made salty? It is no longer good for anything, but to be thrown out and walked on by people."*

This somewhat enigmatic verse holds so much importance when you recognize what Jesus was declaring on the Mount of Beatitudes when He spoke it. Christians the world over have interpreted this verse in different ways, since salt was seen as and used for different things, ranging from a sign of God's covenant to acting as a purifying and preserving agent. But one way it's interpreted is the way I like to understand its meaning, which is this: I believe Jesus was letting us know that when we aren't walking with Him—when we're not connected with Him—we begin to lose our flavor. We start to lose our light, the light that makes us unique and helps us contribute to the world. The message Jesus was trying to get across to His disciples when He first spoke these words to them was that if they remained true to their Christianity, they would never lose their authority and significance.

As you walk this day, call upon this verse to remember the significance of that connection, and how you're called upon to preserve the good Word and to speak about Jesus as often as possible to let others know of your passion for God.

Offer

If you're not already outspoken about your relationship with God, I encourage you to be as open about your faith as possible at every turn. Not just with believers, but with those of other religions and non-believers as well.

Why share your belief with others, no matter what their religious preference may be? One reason is that speaking about something we're passionate about rejuvenates us. It begins to reignite that passion inside ourselves that may not be as intense as it once was. In other words, the more we talk about what moves us, the more we are reminded about why we are driven by that passion in the first place.

Another reason I encourage it: When you hold in your faith, it sometimes shows where you are in regards to what you believe. As long as you're considerate or not judgmental in any way, owning your faith brings about a sense of authority when you speak about it. You're telling others that this is who you are, and because of that, you take ownership of it. And when you do that, you harness even more power from it.

It's also important because you may help rekindle someone else's desire for God that could be ebbing at that moment. It creates a ripple effect. You may not notice it immediately, but know that you're causing positive ripples in all directions. Your faith belongs out there in the world so that everyone who comes in contact with it can appreciate it and be encouraged by it.

Sleep

Before bedtime—preferably about ninety minutes prior to falling asleep—I want you to take a nice warm bath for about twenty minutes. If that's not possible, then spend that time in the shower or enjoy a nice hot foot soak.[1]

Not only does this help you de-stress and unwind from your week; it's also about heating up your body on purpose. You see, as soon as you come out of the hot bath, your body has no choice but to quickly cool down, causing a drop in your body temperature that tells your body it's time for sleep. That's because your body's temperature acts as sort of a sleep gauge as it rises in the day and lowers at night. Triggering it to drop suddenly helps shift your brain and body into sleep mode so you not only fall asleep faster, but experience a deeper, more fulfilling night of rest.

Exercise

Today is an Acknowledge-Pray-Rest Day to give your body the time to rest and heal from your workouts. You may participate in light activities, but be sure to keep an eye on how hard you challenge yourself on this day.

Nutrition

In most cases, the things we choose to flavor our foods—such as dressings, sauces, sour cream, and margarine—tend to be man-made and filled with artificial ingredients, fat, sodium, and other unhealthy fare. That's why the final Faith-Full Food to consider using from this day forward is sea salt, as well as other natural herbs and spices to add flavor to your meals.

However, you should turn to them only when absolutely necessary, and merely as a substitute for high-calorie, fat-laden, or sodium- or sugar-dense sources. And before using a seasoning, consider this: Why are you choosing to mask the flavor of the foods God has provided you? Try reminding yourself that every food has its own unique taste that's meant to be savored, not smothered or suppressed, a flavor that has existed since God first presented it to us. Minimizing or negating any food's true flavor means you're not tasting it in the way it was always intended to be enjoyed.

That said, exploring natural alternatives to season and sharpen the flavor of food, using ingredients that He has also provided us, is entirely fine. Look for all-natural herbs and spices that never put you at risk of ingesting excess calories and artificial ingredients, and that allow you to discover—not cover—the true taste of the foods that God has given all of us. Here are just a handful that I recommend (because of both their taste and the additional healthy advantages they may offer):

Sea salt or Himalayan salt (neither are processed by man, which is the case with iodized salt, and are terrific natural sources of sodium)

Garlic (this cancer fighter not only boosts the immune system but also reduces your risk of stroke and heart disease[2])

Rosemary (it has antibacterial and antioxidant properties, and its scent may also improve memory[3])

Ginger (renowned for easing the digestive system, it is also an anti-inflammatory and aids in the absorption of essential nutrients)

Cumin (in addition to possibly controlling blood pressure and killing harmful bacteria, it also helps with digestion[4])

Sweet basil and cilantro (both fragrant herbs contain vitamin A and vitamin K)

Fennel (a natural appetite suppressant that is also high in vitamin C)

Oregano (not only is it thought to fight cancer, but this popular spice even kills bad bacteria[5])

Cinnamon (this super-spice lowers both inflammation[6] and blood sugar)

Cayenne pepper and paprika (both contain capsaicin, a compound proven to alleviate aches and pains, as well as boost circulation)

Nutmeg and turmeric (both have pain-relieving and anti-inflammatory properties)

DAY 15 (SUNDAY)

THE THIRD SUNDAY

The Week of Purification (Days 15 through 21)

Over the last seven days, you've elevated yourself by adding certain foods, exercises, and practices that have already begun to improve both your physical body and your spiritual body. But the offerings you performed were equally lifting, so before you start the day, ask yourself:

- Did I give as much as I could in all circumstances? If not, don't be discouraged. Instead be proud of your honesty, and know that these elevating offerings can be repeated at any time.
- Did I brighten someone's day? Think about how many people's lives were touched by your generosity during the past week, and let it give you momentum into the next.
- Do you feel more connected to yourself? Your outlook should feel stronger than the week prior.

Throughout this next week, you'll begin to purify both your physical body and your spiritual body by removing and minimizing certain foods, habits, and other adverse elements that are holding you back.

Concede

Father, the heaviness of my unforgiveness has become too much for me to bear. It's hindering my prayer life and my personal life, and it's preventing me from building a deeper relationship with You. Give me the compassion to forgive myself and those You have asked me to reconcile with. Thank You, Father. Amen.

Honor

On this third Sunday, it's important to remind ourselves of Matthew 6:12:

> *"And forgive us our debts, as we have forgiven our debtors."*

Sometimes we fail to connect with Him not due to lack of effort, but because we hold on to certain things that prevent that relationship from growing. It may be wrongful actions that others have committed against us or the guilt of sinning. It may be the shame we feel for not being strong enough in certain moments of our life. But Jesus talks about how if we hold on to resentment, if we are not willing to forgive, then our prayers will never come to pass. Resentment acts as a barrier and prevents us from being the open vessel that God has called us to be, making it more difficult—or even impossible—for us to be used by God.

You must approach God with a cleansed soul and heart, and that can only happen when you begin to forgive not only those who have wronged you but also yourself. As you remove certain things during this week of purification, you will inevitably wonder how this unhealthy stuff ever found its way into your life—and why it's taken this long to address it. We can often become upset with ourselves for allowing negative things to take root in our lives and for not having the courage to do something about them—until now, that is.

Just try to forgive yourself from this moment on, and know that everyone who moves through Seven Sundays comes into this journey bringing their own unique set of unhealthy decisions. As you progress through this week, you'll discover which poor choices are the hardest for you to limit or purge entirely. Then do this:

- Forgive yourself as you bring each one to light.
- Absolve yourself if you don't have the strength yet to delete certain ones this time through Seven Sundays.
- Finally, praise yourself for the effort you made in trying to do something about your poor choices.

Offer

Today reach out to someone whom you have hurt and make amends. Swallow your pride and acknowledge that you mishandled a particular situation in a way that may have affected someone negatively.

Figuring out who to turn to is easier than you might think. Often the guilt we feel is merely God putting that person on your heart. We all have someone on our hearts, and the sooner we reach out to either reconcile or give them more of us than we were able to give previously, the deeper our relationship with God will go. Because when we don't do something about that feeling, it restricts our ability and capacity to relate to God and hear from Him.

Even if you're a kindhearted person by nature, we are all still human, and there are probably times when we could've shown a better side of ourselves to someone. It's just a matter of asking yourself if there have been any moments when you recognize that you could've been more responsible, patient, empathetic, professional, or courteous.

Sleep

This week, you'll be removing certain things that may be negatively impacting your sleep, but there is nothing to prepare for ahead of time. Today look for differences in how you feel or approach specific moments throughout the day that may be a direct result of working toward a better relationship with sleep:

- Did you wake up feeling refreshed or, even better, without needing an alarm clock?
- Do you find yourself more energized and excited to begin the day ahead?
- Were you more focused at church? Did you step away more in thought than usual?
- Did you feel more engaged in conversations with others?

Exercise

Today is another Acknowledge-Pray-Rest Day. Allow your body to recover from what you accomplished on Days 12 and 13. However, you may walk with Him as long as your Worship Walk doesn't exceed thirty minutes and you maintain a relaxed, comfortable pace. If you wish to spend additional time with Him, I encourage you to spend that time in prayer.

Nutrition

The Faith-Full Foods you've begun to incorporate in your diet were introduced last week for a reason. They not only provide an abundance of nutrients that leave you feeling more satiated, but they also boost your energy levels. These two factors alone help make this week of purification a lot easier, since many times we tend to reach for unhealthy foods as quick fixes to either satisfy our hunger or give us instant energy.

To prepare for the next seven days, I encourage you to look ahead at the nutrition portions of Days 16 through 21. That's because each day, you'll be reducing or removing at least one or two of the following Faith-Less Foods from your diet:

High-calorie drinks

Energy bars (and other instant options)

Drive-thru foods

Imitation foods

Sugar

Artificial sweeteners

Vegetable oil (and other refined oils)

Over-processed meats

White bread (and other refined flour products)

Unhealthy add-ons

These ten Faith-Less Foods are mostly man-made or affected by man, are stripped of nutrients, and are high in sugar, unhealthy fats, and excess calories, which is why it's best to minimize or avoid them throughout your Seven Sundays journey. Many of these aren't foods that God provided us, but instead are foods that have come into existence recently. By removing or reducing them in your diet, you'll be stepping away from what didn't exist in biblical times to make more room for foods that have always existed and were meant for us.

But know this: Throughout this week and for the rest of the journey, you're encouraged merely to do your best to minimize and eliminate these Faith-Less Foods. Just do your best, reflect on what they represent in His eyes, and turn to Him first before turning to any of these foods.

DAY 16 (MONDAY)

Concede

Father, You are my source. You are my provider. You are my protector. I will not advance or make any decisions without seeking Your counsel first. I will harness a light that will be consistent because You are the inspiration that sustains me. I'm all-in. Thank you, Father. Amen.

Honor

Today consider Psalm 118:6–8 before starting your day and turn back to these three verses throughout the day:

> *The Lord is on my side; I will not fear.*
> *What can man do to me?*
> *The Lord is on my side, He is among those who help me;*
> *Therefore I will look on those who hate me.*
> *It is better to take refuge in the Lord*
> *Than to trust in man.*

Many people turn to God as a source of strength only when they feel they need it. They reach out to Him in crisis, instead of seeking His guidance with all decisions in their lives, both great and small. In other words, they call upon Him when they're at their lowest, instead of calling upon Him always.

For me, God is my source for everything in my life, and I harness His strength and energy not only during the darkest of moments but in all moments—the good, the bad, the inconsequential, and the insurmountable. Even with decisions I believe require no guidance at all, turning to God can sometimes provide a clarity I never realized was necessary or even possible.

With everything we do and every choice we make, the first step should always be to ask God if what we're about to do is something that He wants for us. Seeking God's counsel for all decisions this week—and along this journey moving forward—will allow you to make the right choice in both the short and the long term. He will sustain you and give you everything you truly need to get through the day.

Offer

God is the source of all we have, but we can also be a source of good things in the world. When we donate blood, we allow ourselves to become a source by offering something sacred—something directly from ourselves. In that way, it gives us an opportunity to make that same connection to the fact that God is our lifeline.

If possible, set up an appointment to give blood today, but don't donate on this day. You'll need to do that on an Acknowledge-Pray-Rest Day, since you shouldn't exercise for twelve hours after giving blood. And waiting a few days will give you time to tell others what you're doing to see if they want to join you.

If you can't give blood (due to a medical condition or being uncomfortable with the process), you could donate to organizations that assist with this task, such as the American Red Cross or the Armed Services Blood Program. Or ask a friend or family member to donate in your place, then go with them and treat them to lunch afterward as a thank-you. Even though you weren't technically the source, you'll have encouraged someone else to be a source, someone who otherwise may never have considered donating that day.

Sleep

Today I want you to begin to recognize the impact that caffeine, nicotine, and alcohol have on your sleep and rethink their use, especially late in the day. If you don't use any of the above, then consider today a cheat day. But if you do, then here's what to keep in mind.

Caffeine. Having this stimulant less than six hours before bedtime can affect your sleep, so set a curfew on your coffee. That also goes for anything chocolate-based (the darker the color, the more caffeine it contains), certain teas (such as black, white, green, and even some herbal varieties), and pain medications such as acetaminophen, aspirin, and ibuprofen (which may have caffeine as an additive to help boost their effectiveness and how fast they work).

Nicotine. Even though most smokers believe that the habit helps them relax, it actually impairs your ability to sleep. Research has shown that both smokers (and even non-smokers who had consumed a small amount of nicotine) experienced less deep sleep, suppressed REM sleep, and had trouble falling and staying asleep.[1] The good news: the negative effects on sleep eventually wear off once you quit.

Alcohol. Although it may make you sleepy, research has shown that alcohol reduces REM sleep (the most restorative form of sleep), suppresses your ability to breathe correctly, and may cause sleep apnea and insomnia.

––––––

One of the many benefits of Seven Sundays is that you'll be working through many things during your journey, and as a result, you will begin to resolve some of the problems or issues that typically weigh heavily on your mind. As these things start to settle themselves, you may find that the need to turn to specific vices begin to wane. Ideally, my hope is that you'll quit turning to things that are unhealthy for you, but at least this starts the process of pulling their use back at night as much as possible.

Exercise

Today you'll walk outside with Him for twenty to thirty minutes, then do a mini-circuit of all five outdoor exercises back-to-back with no rest in between.

- Start by doing Push-ups for twelve repetitions.
- Next, you'll perform Lunges for twelve repetitions (each leg).
- Next, do the Moving Plank for forty seconds.
- From there, you'll perform Burpees for fifteen repetitions.
- Finally, you'll do Supermans for twenty repetitions.
- Rest for one minute by walking (or standing) in place, then repeat the mini-circuit once more for a total of two circuits.

You have several options on when to do the circuit. You can perform it directly before or after your Worship Walk, or walk ten to fifteen minutes first, perform the circuit, then finish your workout with an additional ten to fifteen minutes of walking.

Nutrition

Today I want you to focus on the idea that God is the source of our energy and life. The more you rely on artificial means of getting energy or nutrition, the fewer opportunities you have throughout the day to experience the energy that comes from knowing that He is always there for you. That's why today the two Faith-Less Foods you'll be eliminating from your diet will be high-calorie drinks (including flavored coffee and lattes, soda, and juices) and energy bars (and other instant meal/snack options).

The good news is that you should already feel more energized all day long by sleeping better, eating healthier, and being spiritually rejuvenated as your relationship with God and others continues to strengthen. You should be experiencing, perhaps for the first time, a natural high that should make it easier to step away from the often-abused, highly caloric, artificial sources of energy many turn to in a pinch.

High-calorie Drinks

You may be reaching for high-calorie drinks for their taste, convenience, or simply to be social. Regardless of the reason, try stepping away from any beverages that are high in calories and not all-natural.

Why does juice fall into this category? Juicing fruits and vegetables may seem healthy, but it's not when compared to eating actual fruits and vegetables. Not only does the juicing process remove most—if not all, in some cases—of a fruit or vegetable's fiber, but liquefying it also makes it easier for whatever nutrients are left to pass through your system faster, so fewer are utilized by your body. Also, it causes all of a fruit or vegetable's natural sugar to hit your system at once, triggering your body to immediately release insulin to help store all that sugar within the body—unfortunately, mostly as body fat.

So what about wine and other alcoholic beverages? Some people aren't aware that alcohol actually contains seven calories per gram, which is more than carbohydrates and protein (four calories per gram) and just under fat (which is nine calories per gram). Alcohol is also quickly absorbed into your bloodstream as sugar, which causes your body to release a burst of insulin, a hormone that can lower how much fat your body burns and raise how much fat it stores.

I've had those of the faith say they are confused by my suggestion for curbing wine, since it has always had a presence throughout the Bible and is technically made from what God has provided us. But the Bible also teaches us moderation, and that lesson can be continuously found throughout it as well. For example, Proverbs 20:1 says: *Wine is a mocker, strong drink a riotous brawler; And whoever is intoxicated by it is not wise.* Another example is Ephesians 5:18, where Paul cautioned believers: *Do not get drunk with wine, for that is wickedness, but be filled with the Spirit and constantly guided by Him.* That said, if your faith allows it, enjoying a celebratory drink is fine, but know that each drink you take contains empty calories that your body will most likely be looking to store as body fat if you don't show restraint.

Energy Bars

Despite popular belief, most energy bars (and other instant meal/snack options) are nothing more than nutrient-fortified candy bars processed with unnecessary sugar, calories, and artificial ingredients. That also goes for most protein bars, which offer the promise of sustained energy and muscle-building protein.

Yes, there are some organic bars available, but what can become a problem for many people is their overconsumption. People believe they're healthy because they're all-natural, and that makes many people assume that more is better, and they consume more calories as a result.

If staying away from both of these types of foods seems impossible, think about this: If you tend to reach for either strictly for convenience, why are you so pressed for time in the first place? What's keeping you from preparing a healthier meal or snack? In other words, reflect on the times when you've turned to them in desperation—and question whether that situation could have been prevented through advance planning and preparation.

But that doesn't mean there won't be days when you need an extra boost of energy immediately—and I understand that. Even on days when you legitimately may not have enough time, there are plenty of healthy choices that are equally convenient and compact to choose from. Here are just a few healthier, all-natural, low-sugar options I would suggest:

A piece of whole-grain bread topped with almond butter

A snack-size can of tuna (packed in water) with whole-grain crackers

An apple, banana, or any piece of fruit and a handful of raw nuts

DAY 17 (TUESDAY)

Concede

Father, I realize that my ways haven't worked in certain areas of my life. I'm tired of being selfish, and always wanting what I don't need and not wanting what I do need. I need a new way. I need a better way. I need You, God. I'm willing to risk losing my old self so that I may gain more of You. Thank You, Father. Amen.

Honor

When all we think about is what we can obtain for ourselves, we can end up left with the least in life. That's what Matthew 16:25 makes us realize if we look closely at its meaning:

> *"For whoever wishes to save his life will lose it, but whoever loses his life for My sake will find it."*

When we're willing to forgo all the pleasures and comforts of earthly life for Christ, we're told that we will enjoy an immortal and eternal life, free from all affliction and full of endless delights. Remember today that what we give, we get back—whether in the form of immediate joy from seeing the difference we have made, or later, in some way only God can orchestrate.

Offer

Today I encourage you to donate money to either a charity or your church—or both, if possible. Finances are one of those major areas in our lives where we tend to cling to what we have, either out of self-interest or lack of faith. Even though God has told us it is good to give to those in need, many people still have a hard time trusting God and understanding that when you help those in need, He will give back to you as well.

If you don't have money to give, then look at a few of those things in your life that you've been blessed with but don't seem to use or appreciate as much as someone else might. Today's offering is about asking yourself: If I give this up, will it affect my life negatively? And if not, could it impact someone else's life positively?

That said, if you doubt your ability to give because you feel you don't have enough for yourself, remember that when we feel the need to both obtain and hold on to possessions, there might be other reasons:

- Are you holding on to something because you want others to know you have it?
- Do you feel that object defines you?
- Does it merely bolster your self-worth? Or does it truly bring you joy?

By looking at what you have with an honest eye, you'll begin to see that you have more to give than you realize—and so many opportunities to make a difference in someone's life.

Sleep

Anything that chemically changes or disrupts the way you sleep is essentially preventing your body from operating in the way it was meant to. That's why if you've been relying on sleep aids to fall asleep faster, you should try to stop. Some can lead to dependency, but even if you're using one that's considered non-addictive, most contain antihistamines that your body quickly learns to tolerate. The upshot is, the longer you take a sleep aid, the less effective it eventually becomes.

If you're concerned that you'll have trouble sleeping if you go cold turkey, remember this: By now, you've already made changes that should be affecting your sleep—changes you may not be noticing because you're not letting yourself witness their effects for yourself. You've already introduced certain habits and elements into your bedroom that are meant to help you relax. You're also exercising more regularly and eating better, both of which can help your body rest more comfortably. Most important, you'll be making even more adjustments over the next three and a half weeks that will make it even easier to fall asleep faster. So trust the process and begin to taper off sleep aids.

If you've been using a sleep aid for at least a few months, you may need to wean yourself off it. Take only half of your usual dosage this week, then cut it to a quarter of your usual dosage after the fourth Sunday. After the fifth Sunday, take only a quarter dosage every other night or every three days. Once Seven Sundays is finished, you can stop taking it altogether.

Exercise

Today you'll move through a circuit of all five indoor exercises back-to-back with no rest in between.

- Start by performing the Double-Pump Shoulder Press for twelve repetitions.
- From there, you'll perform Dips for twelve repetitions.
- Next you will do Squat & Holds for twelve repetitions.
- After that, you will do Step Ups for twelve repetitions (each leg).
- Finally, you'll get on the ground and do Bicycles for twenty-five repetitions.
- Rest for three minutes by walking (or standing) in place, then repeat the mini-circuit once more for a total of two circuits.

This will be the first time you've performed a five-move strength-training circuit two days in a row. Because of that, you may find that you're not as fluid going through the workout due to muscle soreness or mild muscular exhaustion (depending on your fitness level).

Know that what you're feeling is entirely normal. Remind yourself that even though you may not be performing at your absolute best on this day, you're strengthening your body nonetheless—and that's what counts. You're also challenging yourself in a way that your body isn't used to, and you'll see even more of a difference in your physical performance as you move through the Seven Sundays program than someone who might be more conditioned than yourself.

Nutrition

Today you'll try to curb or crush two Faith-Less Foods that are more obvious in how they affect our health: drive-thru foods (or fast food of any type) and imitation foods (such as processed cheese, margarine, non-dairy creamer, bacon bits, and butter sprays).

Just the word *imitation* alone should make you question why you would want to eat these types of foods. Whenever we attempt to change, alter, or re-create food that was already perfectly provided for us, the end result is rarely healthier than the original. In most cases, the process tends to remove some (if not all) of the nutrients that God initially placed within the food, and instead exposes us to a variety of man-made chemicals and ingredients that in most cases have proven to be harmful to our health.

That's because many of the additives placed in food to act as sweeteners, preservatives, or artificial dyes are simply used to create a certain texture, flavor, color, or thickness. They don't make food healthier for your body; they simply make it more aesthetically pleasing, less perishable, and harder to resist. In fact, most highly processed foods are also stripped of fiber and nutrients, so even if you're eating what should be healthy for you, it most likely has less of what your body needs and craves.

Finally, keep in mind that every bad meal you consume that breaks your body down takes the place of a healthy meal that could build your body up. It comes down to simple math—the more you rely on fast foods, the fewer opportunities you allow yourself to eat foods that both help and heal you in the way God intended.

Another thing to consider this day is why you're reaching for fast foods in the first place.

Is It a Craving?

Remind yourself that many of the additives in these types of foods (mainly sugar and salt) are put there for that very reason—to make you crave them. You're indirectly being manipulated by your meal. Healthy foods not only satisfy us but trigger a response that lets our body know that it's had its share. But unhealthy foods can have the opposite effect, making us crave more than we require.

Is It Convenience?

If so, take a closer look at how you plan your day, and think back to the last few times you relied on fast food. Was it because you were away from home and found yourself hungry halfway through your day? If that's the case, try to come up with a solution, such as taking along Faith-Full Foods in a cooler or searching for healthier places to eat around an area where you'll be that day.

Is It Economics?

Most people believe that fast food is cheaper, when in reality, home-cooked or home-prepared meals can be just as inexpensive, if not less expensive, overall.

Is It an Emotion?

Sometimes we desire certain foods or flavors because they trigger certain moments from our past. Are those French fries hard to resist because they taste good . . . or do they just remind you of when you were a kid? If you ever find yourself thinking about the past when pulling up to the drive-thru window, finding alternative ways to capture those memories that aren't food-based will serve you better.

Is It Really Saving You Anything in the Long Run?

If leading a healthier lifestyle is your goal, the extra calories and unhealthy fats commonly found in these foods only mean you'll end up spending more time exercising or watching your diet later. The excess sodium widely used as a preservative also means your body will spend more time working harder due to high blood pressure or other health-related issues caused by a high-sodium diet. In other words, if you want to save time, spend more time away from these Faith-Less Foods.

DAY 18 (WEDNESDAY)

Concede

The world distracts me from You, Father. When I get caught up in the world, I become like a leaf blowing in the wind. I wander aimlessly and began to take my focus off You. I will redirect my gaze upon You so that You can help me regain my purpose on this day. Thank You, Father. Amen.

Honor

We can become distracted by our environment. We are bombarded by what's happening around us every waking second of our lives, and it's easy to allow those external circumstances to affect the way we feel and react. But as Romans 12:2 tells us:

> *And do not be conformed to this world, but be transformed and progressively changed by the renewing of your mind, so that you may prove what the will of God is, that which is good and acceptable and perfect.*

The outside world may take our focus off God, but in these verses, Paul talks about how we can be transformed and renewed when we seek the will of God.

Even though living distraction-free is probably impossible, it's important to learn how to live among the chaos of the world—and the key is staying connected to God. When we gaze upon Him during chaotic times, we remain consistent, we are less distracted, and we experience fewer downs and more ups. Through remaining united with Him, you will ultimately be more balanced in every aspect of your life.

Offer

As Christians, we're likely to join a good cause, but how often do you initiate one? Most of us tend to wait for someone else to make the first move. But this time, you will be the first to act. You will make yourself proactive instead of merely reactive. Today look for as many opportunities as possible where you might be able to lead by example.

Finding a situation in which you can be the first to react can be as easy as thinking about what everyone is talking about but no one is doing anything about. Think about something you wish someone would do—and then do it.

For example, think about performing some type of good deed or recognizing something that needs to be fixed or resolved. Look around your town, workplace, school, or home and see if there's a need that no one has noticed yet, or that the community has merely left ignored. You could address a concern you have about someone close to you, or maybe you could just rush toward the door all day long to be the first to open it for others.

By initiating a good work—and not waiting for someone else to take it on—you'll be starting something that is certain to make a positive impact on the world.

Sleep

Avoiding certain foods in the hours before bedtime can help you sleep better. On Day 16, you learned about avoiding chocolate-based foods in the evening hours, but today I want you to consider avoiding spicy and acidic foods as well. You should also avoid going to bed with a full stomach, even if you've only eaten Faith-Full Foods.

Having spicy or acidic fare before bedtime can cause you to have difficulty swallowing, may give you heartburn, and may also contribute to respiratory problems and difficulty breathing[1]—symptoms that can be exacerbated by having a full stomach[2] and lying flat. Even if you don't notice any trouble falling asleep, these potential sleep disruptors could be affecting how you sleep, leaving you feeling more sluggish in the morning.

If you still need to eat something before bedtime, there are smarter ways to curb your hunger without hurting your sleep:

Keep It Smart. Avoid anything with unhealthy fats or added sugars, which can spike your energy and make it difficult to sleep.

Keep It Small. Too many calories before bedtime will cause your body to store them. Make sure your snack is 100 to 150 calories max.

Keep It Stable. Having a snack that combines complex carbohydrates with protein (or a few healthy fats) will keep your blood sugar level throughout the night. Some good examples: a small pear with a tablespoon of peanut butter, one serving of cottage cheese and a handful of berries, or three or four whole-grain crackers and a slice of fresh turkey or chicken.

Exercise

Today is an Acknowledge-Pray-Rest Day. Allow your body to recover from what you accomplished on Days 16 and 17, and skip the strength training. However, if you want to walk with God today, you may do so as long as your Worship Walk doesn't exceed thirty minutes and you maintain an easy, comfortable pace. If you wish to spend additional time with Him, I encourage you to spend that time in prayer to allow your body to recover and heal.

Nutrition

The Faith-Less Food you will try to curb or crush today is sugar, a carbohydrate that is behind many of the highs and lows we experience throughout the day. As you ingest it, sugar causes a release of the feel-good hormone dopamine, which (among other reactions) boosts your energy and concentration. But because sugar is absorbed quickly by your body, that boost doesn't last long, and you reach for more sugary foods over and over again to re-create that feeling.

We all need to take sugar seriously because it's not merely over-consumed in this country; it's also behind everything from obesity, diabetes, and cancer to high blood pressure, kidney stones, and osteoarthritis. That's why as you eat throughout the day, it's a good idea to take a peek at the label of the foods you're consuming to see how many grams of sugar are hiding away in each serving.

Experts recommend that your sugar intake be less than 5 percent of your daily calorie intake: about twenty-four grams for women,[3] although men can have about thirty-six grams.[4] Sadly, most of us eat around three times that amount because, well, it tastes good. That and the fact that it's added to many foods for flavor—even those you wouldn't generally associate with sugar, such as granola, salad dressing, coleslaw, and even ketchup.

If you struggle with eating too much sugar, the first thing to re-mind yourself is that added sugar is filled with calories that contain few to no nutrients. Second, the more you wean yourself from sugar, the more you will taste the natural sugar in the foods He has provided for you.

Within a matter of weeks, the naturally occurring sugars found in dairy products, fruits, vegetables, nuts, and whole grains become more prominent and taste as God intended them to. That's why I'm a firm believer in satisfying sugar cravings through fruit, and I've no-ticed this works with many of my clients too. When my clients eat more fruit, they don't crave as much sugar throughout the day—and you won't either.

DAY 19 (THURSDAY)

Concede

Father, reveal to me what's not honest. Show me the truth about myself and the people in my life. Your Word says that the truth will set me free, so I ask You to set me free from whatever is fake in my life and help me attract more of what is real and authentic. Thank You, Father. Amen.

Honor

Today contemplate John 14:6.

> Jesus said to him, "I am the Way and the Truth and the Life; no one comes to the Father but through Me."

One reason many people fail on their journey is that they aren't confident of the right path to follow. After all, with so many differing opinions out there, each contradicting the other and claiming to be the "easiest" way, discovering the real truth can be difficult, if not impossible.

But the truth is, we know in our hearts that if something is described as the easiest way, it most likely isn't as easy as it sounds or as effective as promised. We already know the right path to follow but shy away from it because we know it may require more time than we want to give or more effort than we may be willing to make.

When you read the Scripture, you realize that we've been shown the right path and that taking it will be fruitful and allow you to experience a higher level of understanding. However, we're also told the truth—that it won't be easy, but it will be rewarding.

The journey you're taking may not be the easiest at times, but know that it is a path that is fulfilling, one where you will experience many victories—both great and small—along the way.

Offer

Do you know the name of every person you see or speak to on a regular basis?

Many of us know people we come into contact with daily but have never bothered to find out their name. It could be that parent at the bus stop, the barista that serves you each morning, your postal carrier, or the person you make small talk with on occasion on the elevator. There is always one person we acknowledge with a nod or a "Hi," but if asked their name, we would come up short. Today you will change that by acknowledging everyone you see by name. If you don't know their name, ask. By making this effort, you're no longer pretending to care—you're showing that you care enough to recognize the person you're speaking to.

If you're worried about being embarrassed for not remembering someone's name, just remember this: the effort of asking shows both humility and respect, and in many cases, it may even open up another level of communication with that individual. You'll be surprised to find that very few people are ever offended that you've taken the time to ask, because it shows how sincere you are about knowing them on a personal level.

Sleep

For some people, a visible clock in the bedroom can serve as an anxiety increaser. Watching time pass can cause you to do math in your mind that can be counterproductive. The dread of having the night hours slip away from you can sometimes create restlessness in certain people, which only exacerbates the problem.

So tonight turn the clock so that it's removed from view, so that if you can't sleep, your curiosity about the time doesn't create or compound your problem. If you use your phone to wake up, place it away from the bed so that it's not easily within reach. This simple act keeps your nervous system in check by reducing the sudden bursts of stress that can occur with each passing glance.

One trick that can help: whenever you feel the need to know the time, try picturing a calm and happy moment in your life instead. Research has shown that using imagery distraction can help you fall asleep twenty minutes faster by clearing unwanted concerns and replacing them with thoughts that are less worrisome.[1]

Exercise

Today you'll Worship Walk for thirty minutes, then hike, bike, or swim—whichever activity you're most comfortable with—for twenty minutes (preferably outdoors, but using a stationary bike, treadmill, or indoor pool is fine if that's your only option).

If none of these options are possible, then you may perform a walk/jog workout instead of hiking, biking, or swimming. To do it: start by walking at a leisurely pace for one to two minutes, then jog for thirty to forty-five seconds. Continue to alternate between walking and jogging for the duration of the workout (twenty minutes total).

Nutrition

Today one of the two Faith-Less Foods you'll be avoiding will be artificial sweeteners. Sugar substitutes can be tempting, since they don't raise your blood sugar or trigger the release of insulin. But even those made from natural sources (such as stevia leaf extract) are still man-made and come with a variety of unhealthy side effects, ranging from decreasing healthy gut bacteria and slowing down your metabolism to contributing to insulin resistance and even making certain medications less effective.

Also, God designed our bodies so that when we crave certain foods, it's because our bodies need the specific nutrients those foods contain. But artificial sweeteners inhibit that natural reaction and make it difficult to listen to our body's needs. They send the wrong message, causing us to crave foods that our bodies not only have no use for, but foods that can be harmful to us when eaten in excess.

The other Faith-Less Food to rethink is vegetable oil (and other refined oils). Not all types of vegetable oil are created equal, and when they are partially hydrogenated or hydrogenated, you're eating an unsaturated fat (molecularly altered by man) that raises your levels of bad LDL cholesterol and lowers your levels of good HDL cholesterol.

Instead, starting today, avoid using any oils with the words *hydrogenated* or *partially hydrogenated* and switch to healthier monounsaturated oils (such as olive, avocado, or canola oil).

DAY 20 (FRIDAY)

Concede

Father, I surrender to Your ways. I know the refining process is meant to strengthen me. Give me hope and perspective during this time so that I may see the light at the end of the tunnel. I don't want to lose my hope and fall short of the metamorphosis. Entrust me with wisdom so that I can make the right use of it. Thank You, Father. Amen.

Honor

God moves through us so that we will become a more improved version of ourselves at the other end—but that happens only when we allow that refinement to take place. The importance of refining can be felt in Zechariah 13:9.

> And I will bring the third part through the fire,
> Refine them as silver is refined,
> And test them as gold is tested.
> They will call on My name,
> And I will listen and answer them;
> I will say, 'They are My people,'
> And they will say, 'The Lord is my God.'

We aren't tested by God because He is unkind or inattentive, but because He knows that when we pass through certain situations, we can become better people—who are more reliant on Him—at the other end. That is why it's vital to understand that through this journey, you're being refined, and that process takes both hard work and patience.

The refinement of any precious metal, such as gold or silver, is never instantaneous nor effortless. The impurities separated from the ore cannot all be removed at the same time. We are the same, in that it takes time for certain bad habits to leave us. Just remember that over time, you'll begin to separate even more from what is bad for you as you start to embrace what is right for you. It requires perseverance and consistency, but that extra effort will make what is left over so unique and valuable—and that's you.

Offer

My hope is that your life is filled with people who care about you, honest and loving people who help you grow and always support you, no matter what. Yet I've also seen many Christians not love themselves enough to say, "This person isn't healthy for me." Continuously pouring effort into someone who isn't trying or giving back in the same way prevents you from putting that same energy into someone who cares enough to work on the relationship you have with them.

God wants what is good for us, but sometimes we may ignore an issue with someone who is negatively affecting our spirit because we're either not strong enough to address the problem or feel guilty for doing so. But today you'll begin to refine your relationships.

Don't worry—we're not just going to start cutting people from your life. Instead I encourage you to take the healthy approach: Explain to this person what's going on in your heart and what you feel needs to change between the two of you. Approach them humbly and in good faith. From there, whatever happens is in God's hands, but you'll have done what you need to do to express how you truly feel.

If that person reacts in a way that shows they're willing to listen and work on the problem, then you know that person is meant to be in your life. But if they aren't in a place to listen to you—or aren't receptive to what you have to say—then it may be necessary to step away from that person (for now) until they reach that place within themselves.

Sleep

The tension we hold in our physical bodies is frequently a reflection of the stress weighing on our spiritual bodies. Releasing that pressure in a way that leaves us physically relaxed can help to ease the burden on our spirit that could be preventing us from falling asleep.

Tonight try a technique known as progressive muscle relaxation, which is as simple as tensing (or flexing) certain muscles and then relaxing them. This simple method has been shown to release built-up tension in a way that places the body in a more relaxed state.

Once you're lying in bed, begin by tensing the muscles in your feet for a minimum of five seconds, relax for twenty seconds, and repeat. (Don't worry if you lose count. Don't focus on numbers, but the feeling. As you go, concentrate on each group of muscles after you relax them.) Keep working your way up your body—through your calves, thighs, posterior, lower back, upper back, chest, shoulders, the back of your arms (triceps), the front of your arms (biceps), forearms, and fingers; then finish with your neck.

When you intentionally focus on portions of your body in this way, you get a better understanding of what your body is feeling in that moment. By tensing each muscle and then allowing it to relax, you'll instantly notice that the relaxed sensation that comes over your muscles affects you spiritually as well, which is why this exercise is just as effective for relaxing the mind as it is for calming the body.

Exercise

Today you'll move through a circuit of all five indoor exercises, performed back-to-back with no rest in between.

- Start by performing the Double-Pump Shoulder Press for twelve repetitions.
- From there, you'll perform Dips for twelve repetitions.
- Next, you will do Squat & Holds for twelve repetitions.
- After that, you will do Step Ups for twelve repetitions (each leg).
- Finally, you'll get on the ground and do Bicycles for twenty-five repetitions.
- Rest for three minutes by walking (or standing) in place, then repeat the mini-circuit twice more for a total of three circuits.

Nutrition

Today the two Faith-Less Foods to minimize or eliminate will be processed meats (this also includes factory-farmed meat and seafood), as well as white bread (and any refined flour product, including pasta made from white flour, as well as white rice).

In both cases, these Faith-Less Foods are examples of refinement gone wrong. Instead of stripping away what is bad for us, these types of foods remove what is healthy (nutrients and fiber, for example) and add in what is not (such as sugar, excess sodium, and artificial ingredients). Also, refined grains are quickly converted into simple sugars that absorb quickly into your bloodstream, creating a blood sugar spike that causes you to store excess fat.

Like many of the Faith-Less Foods, these man-altered versions only exist to make something last longer than God intended it to last or to create a cheaper version of what He wished for you. Going forward, don't settle for less than what was meant for you.

DAY 21 (SATURDAY)

Concede

Father, I thank You for the pruning process. I thank You for cutting off the distractions that inhibit my progress and allowing what is good for me to grow deeper roots. God, let this process teach me to be a better steward so that I can begin to bear good fruit in my life. Thank You, Father. Amen.

Honor

In John 15:1–6, Jesus speaks about how when we remain in God, we grow—and when we are separated from Him, we wither and die:

> *"I am the true Vine, and My Father is the vinedresser. Every branch in Me that does not bear fruit, He takes away; and every branch that continues to bear fruit, He prunes, so that it will bear more fruit. You are already clean because of the word which I have given you. Remain in Me, and I in you. Just as no branch can bear fruit by itself without remaining in the vine, neither can you unless you remain in Me. I am the Vine; you are the branches. The one who remains in Me and I in him bears much fruit, for apart from Me you can do nothing. If anyone does not remain in Me, he*

is thrown out like a branch, and withers and dies; and they gather
such branches and throw them into the fire, and they are burned."

Many times, we make our lives more chaotic simply because we feel that if we're not multitasking, we're either behind the curve or missing out on something. We add and keep many branches—even the ones that bear no fruit—because we believe it makes us a better person. Or we keep ourselves busy because it distracts us from addressing something we could be putting more effort into: our relationship with God, with others who love us, and even the relationship we have with ourselves.

Simplifying our lives lets us focus our attention on Him and all the blessings He has bestowed upon us. It allows us to recognize which things in our lives bear no fruit and take us away from serving Him, to be there for those we love, and to love ourselves.

Today think about these verses and look for those branches in your own life. Then begin the pruning process by either reprioritizing or re-moving what may be overcomplicated in your life in either unhealthy or unproductive ways.

Offer

Today all I ask is that you say "Thank you" as often as possible—in fact, at every imaginable opportunity. Ask yourself if there's an oppor-tunity to thank everyone you meet for something, and if so, look that person in the eye and smile when you do it. Even if you had thanked them previously, just do it again—because a "Thank you" is never wasted.

This offering may seem small, but its power to positively change the world is often underestimated. When you say "Thank you," it's an immediate sign of appreciation and respect. You are acknowledging someone for what they have done for you, which (if you're thanking them) was something either kind or of value. It also rewards that person by making them feel proud about their considerate act. That alone might encourage them to continue their kindness, making your "Thank you" a motivating force behind other possible acts of thoughtfulness they might perform afterward.

Finally, if you doubt the power of saying "Thanks" at every possible moment, ask yourself this: How many times have you heard someone dwell on how they had wished someone would have thanked them for something they did? You might have even been this person at some point.

How did it feel? Did not hearing those words make you feel less significant or appreciated? Would you be less inclined to help that individual again, remembering that they hadn't thanked you previously? Recall that feeling and remember that you can create the exact opposite effect on someone's spirit using two simple words.

Sleep

Falling behind in the littlest of things can set the tone for the rest of our day. That's why you'll begin making your bed this morning—and every morning from now on.

Just seeing a task—one that shouldn't take more than a few seconds—unfinished serves as proof that we began the day rushed. Seeing it can make you feel incapable of handling the simplest of tasks. It becomes yet another example of something you had to do but decided to ignore.

Making your bed may seem inconsequential, but doing it brings a certain amount of comfort into your life. Making your bed is that first obstacle of the day—that first opportunity to show yourself that you'll get done what needs to get done. It's proof first thing in the morning, before you even start your day, that you're on top of your life. If you don't make your bed regularly, start doing so today.

Exercise

Today is an Acknowledge-Pray-Rest Day. Allow your body to recover from what you accomplished on Days 19 and 20 by forgoing any form of strength-training exercise. However, if you want to walk with God on this day, you may do so as long as your Worship Walk doesn't exceed thirty minutes and you maintain a relaxed, comfortable pace. If you wish to spend additional time with Him, I encourage you to spend that time in prayer to allow your body to recover and heal.

Nutrition

Your final Faith-Less Food to either lessen or lose on this day (and moving forward): the use of unhealthy add-ons.

This goes back to simplifying your life and looking at the branches that aren't yielding any fruit. Sour cream, sauces, condiments, dressings, gravies, and many of the things we pour or spread onto our foods to add additional flavor also tend to add excess calories, fat, sugar, and other ingredients with no nutritional value. Today look at each add-on as a branch, and remind yourself that if it's not making what you're eating healthier, then it's a branch that deserves to be trimmed or cut.

I get it. For some people, this may be the hardest change to make. But when certain foods lack a little zest and you simply have to add something to make a Faith-Full Food more flavorful, here are a few tricks (and compromises) you can try:

- Replace your dressing or sour cream with a little salsa, lemon juice, or a tiny dollop of low-fat or nonfat Greek yogurt.
- Make your own dressing using a little lemon juice, a little olive oil, and some Himalayan salt and pepper.

- Instead of using spaghetti sauce, throw on some chopped tomatoes with a hint of fresh basil and a dash of olive oil.
- Season things up with herbs and spices, such as chili powder, dill, rosemary, or tarragon. They're calorie-free and add plenty of flavor, without any of the sugar, cholesterol, or fat you would expect from most unhealthy add-ons.
- If giving up this Faith-Less Food category is impossible, then measure out what you typically would throw onto your food and take away a quarter to a half of what you would normally have.

DAY 22 (SUNDAY)

THE FOURTH SUNDAY

The Week of Adaptation
(Days 22 through 28)

The act of purification isn't easy, especially if many unhealthy things have found a home in our lives. How far you've come up to this point, particularly with your nutritional habits, is up to you as you walk with Him. But along the way—and especially today—keep this in mind:

- If the past seven days were difficult for you, that's normal. This is a journey, not a set path, and all you have to do is try your best. And if your best at this point isn't what you want it to be, remember that you have the power to change that.
- Even if you managed to minimize or remove only one Faith-Less Food, you are further along than you were the week before.
- If you managed to substitute only one Faith-Full Food for a Faith-Less Food, be thankful that you are further along than you were the week before.

That said, during this week of adaptation, you will take many of the things you've learned and set healthier limits for yourself. Too much of anything in our lives—even when those things are good for us—may keep us from becoming a more well-rounded person both inside and out. It's when we're in a state of equilibrium that we're most able to flourish.

This week, we'll work on creating a rhythm by bringing balance to your prayer life, your sleep schedule, your relationship with food, and time spent at work and with family—among other things—so that you may also spend more time with Him.

Concede

Father, the balance I yearn for and envision will first require that You be at the center of my life. I ask You to help me connect the dots beyond that. Show me the areas in my life where I need to focus more of my attention and allow me to see the areas that require less attention. Help make things practical for me so that I can begin to create some type of rhythm in my life. Thank You, Father. Amen.

Honor

Taking the time to find the right levels with everything in our lives is so crucial, but it all starts with Him, as Matthew 6:33 reminds us:

> But first and most importantly seek His kingdom and His righteousness, and all these things will be given to you also.

We create so much imbalance in our lives because often we want more of this or that. Pursuing things to excess, rather than seeking God, creates extremes in some regions of our lives and leaves voids in others. But God tells us that if we place Him in the center, all the other things in our lives will fall into place as they should. God will help us prioritize our lives, but He can only help us if we make an effort to seek Him out first.

Offer

Do you trust God enough to let an opportunity or credit pass to someone else equally worthy or deserving? Do you feel confident that if you allow someone else to go through this door, God will open another one for you? Is there something being handed to you right now that you could either share with or give to someone else who deserves it equally?

Today look for the person who may not be getting the break or attention they deserve, whether at work, within your circle of friends, within your church, or even in your household. Seek out that person who always seems to be passed by for the merit they deserve, then make sure they get it today.

Try to mention those who deserve praise as often as possible. Instead of directing attention toward yourself in conversation, think of ways to outwardly project appreciation toward others. Often when we bring someone's name up in conversation, it's to gossip about them, not to glorify them. But today spread the good news about other people's acts of kindness, talents, and positive personalities when they're not present.

Sleep

Over this next week, you won't be asked to bring in anything new or take anything away when it comes to your sleep environment, so there's nothing to prepare for. Instead you'll spend the next seven days bringing balance to your sleep habits in simple ways. Every day or so, you'll consider how you approach sleep in certain ways that may allow both your physical body and your spiritual body to relax even more efficiently.

Exercise

Today is another Acknowledge-Pray-Rest Day. Allow your body to continue recovering from Days 19 and 20. You may walk with Him for up to thirty minutes at an easy, comfortable pace, but if you have been experiencing difficulty with the exercise portion of Seven Sundays, rest on this second day in a row and spend that time in prayer instead.

Why? Because this week, your workouts will begin to get more intense to challenge you even further. However, if at any time the routine seems too intense, you can scale it back accordingly.

Nutrition

This week, there is nothing to prepare for nutritionally because you won't be changing what you eat—but *how* you eat. So today consider the following:

- How do you decide how much food to put on your plate?
- Do you eat only when hungry—or at specific times of the day?
- Is dinner typically your final meal of the day?
- Do you tend to skip meals when the day gets away from you?

I pose these questions merely to make you aware of your eating habits before showing you a smarter way to enjoy the foods He has provided for you. So today merely reflect on these thoughts.

Also, with the addition of Faith-Full Foods and the elimination of Faith-Less Foods in place, you're now moving toward eating only what He has provided us. However, the reason most people struggle with their diets is that they assume that if they don't make *every* single change, or if they occasionally fall into temptation, then they have failed.

A lot of people quit when they feel they can't do something with 100 percent effort. Yet who among us is ever able to lead a perfect Christian life? When we sin or stray from the path, it's natural to lament and condemn ourselves. Yet we accept that He understands that hiccups are a natural part of our salvation, that despite how often we stumble, He still loves us and always allows us to try again and continue.

When it comes to eating healthy, we don't allow ourselves that forgiveness. Being 100 percent all-in with your diet is terrific, but don't let mistakes discourage you. In other words, it's natural to be scared that you're going to slip—and upset with yourself when you do—but when that happens, keep in mind that God never expects perfection but encourages faith. So have faith in yourself moving forward, try your best, be proud of what you've achieved, and forgive yourself for the things you've wrestled with for now.

DAY 23 (MONDAY)

Concede

Father, I want to start seeing my life with Your perspective. I often overlook what's good and what I should be grateful for. This sometimes leads me to not see the truth in my life, and often I begin to feel bad about my situation. Change my lens, Father, so that I can start seeing my life differently and to be grateful for what I do have. Thank You, Father. Amen.

Honor

On this first day of adaptation, consider Isaiah 55:8–9.

> *"For My thoughts are not your thoughts, nor are your ways My ways," declares the Lord. "For as the heavens are higher than the earth, so are My ways higher than your ways and My thoughts higher than your thoughts."*

It's so easy to get caught up in the way others believe, even when we know we should—and can—approach things differently. These two verses remind us that we must strive to share the same outlook as God, for when we attempt to follow His perspective, the decisions we make will always remain wiser and purer than when we allow the world to shape our thoughts.

Sometimes simply switching our perspective has an immediate effect on our actions. Those of faith don't always think like the world thinks or see things as the world sees them. Instead we try to approach things from a devout viewpoint based on our belief and on God's Word. So, from this point forward, choose His ways and think His thoughts—and see how those simplest of actions can take you further than you ever imagined.

Offer

Today I want to encourage you to stop doing something that I hope isn't an action you take part in anyway—gossiping about others.

We don't always gossip because we're bitter about or jealous of another person, though sometimes that is the reason. Often it's because we have nothing better to talk about. Gossip becomes a conversation filler that prevents us from exploring a deeper relationship with the person we're speaking to. Every minute wasted talking negatively about someone else is a minute you could have spent getting to know the person you're speaking with. Replace gossip with grace, and try to only speak words that add value to a person's life instead of words that don't match the ways and thoughts of God.

We're not always aware of the circumstances surrounding all the people in our lives, and we can't always be certain that everything we hear about someone is entirely accurate. But even if it is, you're not helping that person change into someone better by talking behind their back. The only thing you're changing is someone's perspective about that individual in an unflattering way.

We all have our good and bad moments. We are all capable of committing actions that are righteous and actions that are wrong. By spreading gossip, you're not only keeping someone's bad moment alive, but you're possibly hurting that person by prejudicing others against them.

I also encourage you to stop those around you from gossiping as well. Doing this ensures that the person you're speaking to is also able to spend more quality time with you, but there's also a bigger reason. Each time you close down a conversation rooted in gossip before it starts, it makes the gossiper rethink their actions, not just in that moment, but later on when they're tempted to gossip to someone else. It may make them reconsider their negative words by making them more aware that what they're doing isn't something looked at favorably by all.

Sleep

We each operate differently from one another, which is why it's important to listen to our bodies, particularly after exercise. Most of us become energized after we work out because of the physical changes that occur. Our body temperature rises, our heart rate increases, and our body releases adrenaline, which makes us more alert.

But because I'm not certain at what point in the day you've been working out, I need you to consider this: some people who exercise before going to bed never experience trouble sleeping and may in fact find drifting off much easier. But there are also some who find it harder to fall asleep. If that's you, then you might want to reconsider when you exercise, especially if it could be affecting your quality of sleep.

Exercise

Today you'll walk outside with Him for twenty to thirty minutes, then do a mini-circuit of all five outdoor exercises back-to-back with no rest in between.

- Start by doing Push-ups for fifteen repetitions.
- Next, you'll perform Lunges for fifteen repetitions (each leg).
- Next, do the Moving Plank for fifty seconds.
- From there, you'll perform Burpees for fifteen repetitions.
- Finally, you'll do Supermans for twenty-five repetitions.
- Rest by jogging (either in place or forward) for five minutes, then repeat the circuit once more for a total of two circuits.

As always, you can perform the circuits directly before or after your Worship Walk, or walk ten to fifteen minutes first, perform the circuit, then finish your workout with an additional ten to fifteen minutes of walking.

Nutrition

Most people don't have to eat as much food as they might think. I often see people choose healthy foods, but then overindulge. They then become confused about why they still struggle with their weight, even though they're eating nothing but Faith-Full Foods. But once I look at how much healthy food they're consuming throughout the day, the problem becomes exceedingly apparent.

By gaining a better perspective on the right portion sizes—the proper amount of food that your body was designed to break down efficiently—you'll find yourself eating less yet feeling satisfied. To make sure you're never consuming more food than required according to God's design, try using the following tactics to measure your food at each meal or snack:

- A three-ounce serving of cooked chicken, fish, or meat is the size of a deck of cards (or a woman's palm).
- A one-cup serving of whole-grain pasta or rice (cooked) is the size of a tennis ball.

- A one-ounce serving of nuts, pretzels, or chips is roughly one handful.
- A one-ounce serving of cheese is the size of two pairs of dice.
- An average single serving of fruit or vegetables is the size of a tennis ball.
- A single serving of green salad is the size of an open-cupped hand.
- A standard-sized baked potato is the size of a baseball.
- A teaspoon-sized serving of fats, oils, or butter is the size of the tip of your thumb.
- A healthy single serving of salad dressing is the size of your thumb.

Adjusting to these portion sizes may be difficult at first; you may have your body to blame for giving you the wrong perspective. If your body has been trained up to this point to overconsume, you may have been teaching your body to believe it needs more food than it truly does. Your body may tell you at first that it requires larger portion sizes than you're allowing it to have.

But don't worry: Very soon—you must have faith about this—your body will adjust. Your stomach will begin to shrink after you introduce these new portion sizes. It's a process that takes patience. Learning this perspective for the first time is not necessarily an easy change for most people, but your body will eventually adapt and return to how it was always designed to function—as God intended it to function.

DAY 24 (TUESDAY)

Concede

Father, how do you want me to spend my day? Show me how to value my time. I don't mean that in a worldly way, in which I'm hustling from one place to another, but in a godly way, where I'm trusting Your timing and allowing the Spirit to guide my steps. Thank You, Father. Amen.

Honor

The value of time is something to consider as you read Ephesians 5:15–16:

> *Therefore see that you walk carefully, not as the unwise, but as wise, making the very most of your time, because the days are evil.*

The life we're living is the only one we get, yet when people think on this point, it reminds many that they have to work, achieve, or earn more. Most people tend to think about all the things and experiences they need to obtain; they look at time in a worldly way.

When we're continually hustling, we may *feel* we're getting a lot done, but we're not filling ourselves up emotionally and spiritually.

We get so distracted by constantly racing toward the next goal or thing that we're less available to the people around us.

Yet when we're productive doing only what God has called us to do, and when we're present in the moment, it raises us emotionally and spiritually. It grants us pause to appreciate those around us and gives us the breather we need to look more closely at what it is we're so desperate to obtain. If you will just take a second, you may discover that what you seek is to feel loved, and that love may already be all around you, but you're running right past it.

Offer

There are always people in our lives who cry out for help or just want someone to talk to. Sometimes we may overlook that need or give them less of ourselves because we feel rushed to move on to the *next thing* we have to do. Even when we do take the time to pay attention, we may dwell on that *next thing*, which also detaches us from the present occasion.

But God has called you to be with that person.

That's why today I encourage you to try being present in every encounter and conversation. Instead of putting a time limit on any discussion, let each occur naturally and organically, giving that person more time than you might think you have. It's about being intentionally emotionally available, asking yourself if the person in front of you needs more time with you, and recognizing that their need may be greater than your own.

Sleep

God designed us with a built-in system (known as a circadian biological clock) that regulates how sleepy or awake we feel over a twenty-four-hour period. Our circadian rhythm rises and falls at different times of the day and varies from person to person. Once again, we are all unique according to His design.

But one thing is true for everyone: Establishing a sleep schedule—and being consistent with when you go to bed—allows that internal clock do its job. When you're erratic with your sleep schedule—going to bed and waking up at different times during the week—you prevent your body from establishing a natural sleep cycle.

From this point forward, if you haven't been consistent with your bedtime, try your best to do that. Pick a time to call it quits for the night and a time to wake up, and stick with them—even on the weekends, when you may be tempted to go to bed late and sleep in.

Exercise

Today you'll move through a circuit of all five indoor exercises back-to-back with no rest in between.

- Start by performing the Double-Pump Shoulder Press for fifteen repetitions.
- From there, you'll perform Dips for a total of fifteen repetitions.
- Next, you will do Squat & Holds for a total of fifteen repetitions.
- After that, you will do Step Ups for a total of fifteen repetitions (each leg).
- Finally, you'll get on the ground and do Bicycles for a total of thirty repetitions.
- That's one circuit. Rest for two minutes by walking (or standing) in place, then repeat the mini-circuit twice more for a total of three circuits.

Nutrition

Today you'll take the time to eat at a slower pace. One thing many people forget is that it takes roughly twenty minutes for your stomach to tell your brain that it's full. If you're not careful and eat too quickly at every meal or snack, you can easily find yourself taking in more calories than your body really needs before that signal finally reaches your brain.

I'm not asking you to time yourself. But there are several ways you can extend your mealtime without having to put much thought into it. For example, try chewing your food twenty or thirty times before swallowing it. Other tricks you can try include taking a sip or two of water after every bite or, if you're dining with family and friends, making a point of having a bit of conversation between each bite.

By the way, if certain foods seem almost impossible to chew that many times, chances are they are Faith-Less Foods. You'll begin to notice that healthier Faith-Full Foods tend to have more substance because most are packed with nutrients and fiber that take a little more work to nosh on. I love this meal-lengthening trick for the way it can open your eyes to the difference between the foods God has given us and the foods man makes.

DAY 25 (WEDNESDAY)

Concede

Father, I'm tired of falling short of the mark. Help me to step up my game so that I can be ready for the victory You have in store for me. Open my eyes to the little details so that they become habits in my life. I want to be prepared for the responsibility You put on my life. Thank You, Father. Amen.

Honor

In Matthew 24:44, the Bible reminds us that Christ is coming—and tells us how we must prepare for Him:

> *"Therefore, you must also be ready; because the Son of Man is coming at an hour when you do not expect Him."*

Today we're thinking about the importance of readying ourselves for what's to come. The verse speaks about how, as Christians, we should be getting ready every day for that moment when He arrives.

That same sense of planning is what we should bring to everything in our lives. When we aren't prepared, disorganization can make what we have to accomplish more difficult, more time-consuming, and far more frustrating. It creates chaos that causes us to lose interest in the task at hand, as well as a deeper connection with what we're attempting to do.

But being more on top of things sets us at ease. It keeps us from losing sleep, making poor choices, or skipping certain opportunities that are healthy for us because we lack enough time. In short, it removes much of the chaos that can blur or interfere with us being our best self at that moment—and being closer to God.

Offer

We all know someone who may not have the best handle on a certain circumstance but might be too selfless or embarrassed to ask for help. Someone who could use a little more organization in their life so that they can get more out of life.

Instead of relating to their problem by saying, "I've been there"— today tell them, "I'm here, so how can I help?" Think of this moment as an opportunity to ask if there is any way you can help minimize some of their stress by attacking, with them, whatever problem they have. It's a chance to strip away anxiety and fear from someone's spirit by merely making their day a little less hectic.

You don't have to do much. What you do could be as simple as picking a few things up for them at the store, offering to take their kids to school, or helping them think through a situation for which they may need a second opinion. Just taking one task off their plate may help them out tremendously in a way that brings them back into focus.

Offering assistance may seem bold, and to be honest, it could come off as presumptuous to some. So instead of telling someone that they *look like* they could use a hand, just *ask* if they could use a hand. Or tell them how desperate you are to do something today and how they would be helping *you* by letting you chip in.

Sleep

Bringing your body into the best alignment possible at bedtime may seem insignificant, but it's something that could have a tremendous impact on the quality of your sleep. Tonight try preparing yourself by placing a few pillows in the perfect position—depending on how you typically doze. If you sleep:

- On your back: Place a pillow underneath your knees and stick a rolled-up towel under the small of your back to straighten out your body.
- On your stomach: Put a pillow underneath your hips and stomach—this will raise your middle to keep your spine in line and take stress off your lower back.
- On your side: Bend your knees and tuck a pillow between them to bring your hips and spine into alignment.

Even though you'll most likely shift during the night, you'll still spend a certain amount of time with your body in better alignment, which could enhance the quality of your sleep during those particular hours.

Exercise

Today is an Acknowledge-Pray-Rest Day. Allow your body to recover from what you accomplished on Days 23 and 24 by forgoing any form of strength-training exercise. However, if you wish to walk with God on this day, you may do so as long as your Worship Walk doesn't exceed thirty minutes and you maintain a relaxed, comfortable pace. If you wish to spend additional time with Him, I encourage you to spend that time in prayer to allow your body to recover and heal.

Nutrition

Many of God's creatures are either diurnal (most active during the day) or nocturnal (most active at night). As diurnal creatures, our bodies operate based on the sun, particularly when the sun rises and when it sets. But because He designed us to be highly adaptable, we also have the ability to become nocturnal as well.

Being able to see and function well past sunset can confuse our bodies and keep us craving food long after we need to be eating. That's why I recommend that my clients—and now you—set a food curfew at 8:00 p.m. (or roughly three hours before you usually go to bed) if weight loss is a goal. That doesn't mean you can't have a small snack before bedtime if hunger pangs may affect your sleep. In that case, follow the guidelines set in the Sleep portion of Day 18, which are:

Keep It Smart. No unhealthy fats or added sugars; both boost energy and make it harder to fall sleep.

Keep It Small. Shoot for a snack that delivers 100 to 150 calories at most, so you don't store excess body fat.

Keep It Stable. Making that snack a combination of complex carbohydrates with protein (or a few healthy fats) will keep your blood sugar stable throughout the night.

DAY 26 (THURSDAY)

Concede

Father, let me feel Your wholeness through Your Word and Spirit. I want to submerge myself fully into You. Give me focus to turn in Your direction when my flesh turns weak. I want to find in You the nourishment that comes from Your will and not my own. Thank You, Father. Amen.

Honor

Matthew 4:3–4 reminds us that there's such a thing as spiritual hunger:

> *And the tempter came and said to Him, "If You are the Son of God, command that these stones become bread." But Jesus replied, "It is written and forever remains written, 'Man shall not live by bread alone, but by every word that comes out of the mouth of God.'"*

These two verses explain that we don't simply live off food, but that we also need sustenance of the spirit—and the two are more connected than you might imagine.

Have you ever asked yourself why you may be reaching for certain Faith-Less Foods? Our hunger for a deeper connection with God and others can sometimes cause us to reach for temporary satisfaction through food. When we don't satisfy ourselves spiritually through prayer and fellowship, certain negative emotions, such as fear, self-doubt, and loneliness, can linger and grow stronger. That is when we can be more prone to make less healthy choices to distract or comfort us.

But by feeding the spirit through Scripture and fellowship, you re-center yourself spiritually and begin to find that your temptation to reach for unhealthy foods begins to wane. We can enjoy the kind of nourishment that comes only when we turn that moment over to God and allow Him into that space.

Offer

Today you'll become a part of solving someone else's food issues by fighting hunger in some way. It might be donating to an organization such as Feeding America, the No Kid Hungry program, Save the Children, or World Hunger Relief, Inc. Or it can be as simple as looking locally for schools, churches, and other groups that are collecting food for those in need.

You could also use social media to find out from friends and acquaintances if they're aware of any food drives happening at that moment. The reason I like this approach is that your request may encourage others to do the same or remind them of a food drive they meant to contribute to.

If your contribution is food instead of a monetary donation, I encourage you not to simply reach for the things in your pantry that you might typically pull together. Often people donate the stuff they have no use for or find less desirable. As you collect items, try remembering that you're not only feeding someone, but you're accountable to a certain degree for what they're taking into their bodies.

With that responsibility in mind, consider collecting healthier foods, as well as food items that may bring a smile to their face. Or, if you have the means, consider taking a shopping trip specifically to buy items instead of relying on what's left over in your pantry. Don't use this opportunity just to feed someone; make it a moment to help strengthen and nourish them.

Sleep

Just as we hunger for food, we also hunger for sleep at times when we least expect it. Even though you should be enjoying a more productive, longer, deeper sleep throughout this journey, you may be craving a nap on certain days as the exercise portion of Seven Sundays begins to intensify. That is entirely natural, and listening to your body's need for additional sleep is wise. However, just be sure that you nap the right way so that it doesn't affect your overall sleep during the night.

Even though everyone is different, most experts agree that a nap of between ten and thirty minutes is ideal. Any longer and you risk falling into a deeper sleep that could leave you feeling groggier when you wake up and affect how well you sleep that evening.

Exercise

Today you'll walk outside with Him for twenty to thirty minutes, then do a mini-circuit of all five outdoor exercises back-to-back with no rest in between.

- Start by doing Push-ups for fifteen repetitions.
- Next, you'll perform Lunges for fifteen repetitions (each leg).
- Next, do the Moving Plank for fifty seconds.
- From there, you'll perform Burpees for fifteen repetitions.

- Finally, you'll do Supermans for twenty-five repetitions.
- Rest by jogging (either in place or forward) for five minutes, then repeat the circuit once more for a total of two circuits.

Nutrition

You may have noticed how many of God's Faith-Full Foods—particularly green tea, vegetables, and fruits—are rich in water, which helps hydrate our bodies. But today consider how much additional water you're taking in.

Keeping your body hydrated helps it perform a variety of vital functions, including transporting nutrients and oxygen to your cells, assisting in digestion, regulating your body temperature and blood pressure, and flushing away toxins—among many others. Drinking enough water can also help you feel satiated, which will be extremely important for the weeks ahead when you'll be fasting.

If you prefer exact amounts, try drinking a minimum of sixty-four ounces of water during the day. Ideally, I would love for you to drink even more—up to half your body weight (but convert the pounds to ounces). For example, if you weigh 160 pounds, you could shoot for eighty ounces of water daily. But if you're not the type to keep track, just try a few of these tricks that should keep you hydrated all day long:

- Carry a water bottle with you at all times, or if that's not convenient, place glasses or bottles at various places that you frequent throughout the day. That way, you'll always have something to reach for.
- Once your glass is half empty, fill it back up. The more water you have access to, the more water you'll likely drink during the day.

- If plain water isn't your thing, try infusing it with a few flavorful Faith-Full Foods. Add a few slices of fruit or vegetables (and even individual spices and herbs) to a container of cold water, then let it sit in the fridge for a few hours. Some of my favorite infusion foods are berries, citrus fruits, melons, carrots, cucumber, cinnamon sticks, ginger, mint or basil leaves, and fennel.

DAY 27 (FRIDAY)

Concede

Father, I love that You care about every little desire, joy, worry, and fear that I have in my life. I love the fact that You are in every little detail. It gives me confidence, knowing there's nothing trivial about me. It shows that You care for me more than I could ever imagine. I now want this love to transition into the way that I treat myself and others in my life. Thank You, Father. Amen.

Honor

I've spoken a few times already about how we are created in the image of God, and how He has thought of every detail, which is what Ephesians 2:10 exemplifies:

> *For we are His workmanship, created in Christ Jesus for good works, which God prepared beforehand, so that we would walk in them.*

An artist paints a masterpiece in which every little detail matters and means something. Builders put every bit of their effort and love into an object they're constructing. We were created by God in the same manner. He thought about every little detail within us, and it's not portions of you that He loves—He loves every single thing about you.

In other words, the little things count.

The small decisions we make every day are what allow us to build our relationship with Him, and they're also important when it comes to how we treat ourselves.

I encourage you to look at all the things you do each day on this journey—all the offerings and changes—as a series of little details that collectively express love for yourself.

Everything you're doing, no matter how small—all of these little things add up in the long run. In many ways, this entire journey is about having a different perspective on the tiny things that help make up the big picture, just as He appreciates every single detail about you.

Offer

We tend to only see God during the "big" moments, those life-changing events when it's impossible not to recognize His handiwork. We may glorify His work when we witness a magnanimous sunset, see someone overcome illness, or hold a newborn in our hands. But it's important to remember that His work can be found in everything. Being aware of the "little" moments, the places where God isn't hiding but merely goes unnoticed reminds us that God is present with us always.

Today don't just find Him in the obvious. Look for Him in the smallest of details. Reflect on every nuance of everything and everyone you encounter, and look for His work within. When you're moved emotionally by listening to music, hugging your children, savoring the flavor of a Faith-Full Food, or remembering something that touched you, you're experiencing His work. You'll soon discover that the more you seek out God, the sooner you'll realize that He's easy to find—because He's all around you.

Sleep

Every little thing matters. That fact is never more important than when we bring even the smallest of unresolved issues or frustrated thoughts into the bedroom before sleep. Having something on our hearts that we haven't quite worked through can unconsciously keep us from falling asleep quickly or deeply.

Many times, these matters can be eased by taking a few minutes to address or acknowledge them. On this night and each evening moving forward, try setting a timer two hours before bedtime to remind yourself to ponder this question: Is there anything I need an answer to—or situation I need to take care of—before going to sleep?

Home in on the issues or concerns that are in your mind at that moment. Even if it's something you can't fix or adjust that day, just walking through everything in your mind for a few minutes can help bring resolution. That way, when you approach sleep later that evening, you'll feel more relaxed, knowing that you've either addressed these issues or given them the attention and thought they required.

Exercise

Today you'll move through a circuit of all five indoor exercises back-to-back with no rest in between.

- Start by performing the Double-Pump Shoulder Press for fifteen repetitions.
- From there, you'll perform Dips for fifteen repetitions.
- Next, you will do Squat & Holds for fifteen repetitions.
- After that, you will do Step Ups for fifteen repetitions (each leg).
- Finally, you'll get on the ground and do Bicycles for thirty repetitions.

- Rest for two minutes by walking (or standing) in place, then repeat the mini-circuit twice more for a total of three circuits.

Nutrition

The physical bodies that God has given us are perfectly crafted, but when we go against the way they're meant to operate, we find ourselves in difficulty.

Our bodies were never meant to take in a lot of food at one time. Think about anything in nature, such as a plant or a tree. Watering is essential, but overwatering is detrimental. That's because a plant's roots can absorb only so much at one time. Our bodies are no different, and when we either overeat in one sitting or wait too long between meals, our bodies make adjustments in ways that can slow down our metabolism, cause us to store excess fat, and break down healthy muscle tissue for energy.

But when you place yourself on a food schedule, your body begins to learn and know when it's going to eat next. This helps you feel more satiated and less likely to reach for Faith-Less Foods or to crave more food than your body needs at the moment. It also allows our bodies to operate more efficiently and absorb nutrients more readily, so we utilize more of what God has provided us within our food.

Starting today, have breakfast, then try to have either a healthy meal or snack every two to three hours from that point forward. For example, if you started your day with a 7:00 a.m. breakfast, try something like this:

- Have a snack at 9:30–10:00 a.m.
- Eat lunch at 12:00–12:30 p.m.
- Have another snack at 2:30–3:00 p.m.

- Eat dinner at 5:00–5:30 p.m.
- Have (if needed) a final snack at 7:00–7:30 p.m.

Even if you're the type who wakes up early and gets home late, the same math applies—just adjust things to match your schedule (so long as you're eating something every two to three hours). For example, if you normally can't eat dinner until 7:00, try a schedule such as:

- Eat breakfast at 7:00 a.m.
- Have a snack at 10:00 a.m.
- Eat lunch at 1:00 p.m.
- Have another snack at 4:00 p.m.
- Eat dinner at 7:00 p.m.
- Have (if needed) a final snack at 9:00–9:30 p.m.

DAY 28 (SATURDAY)

Concede

Father, I want to know You more. I want to be able to discern Your voice. Teach me in these times of solitude how to be more like You. Fill me up spiritually, emotionally, and physically so that I can give more to those around me. Thank You, Father. Amen.

Honor

It seems that so many of us never appreciate the strength of solitude. It's as if the prospect of being alone is somehow depressing and immediately needs to be rectified. But it's in those quiet moments that we can aim all our attention toward God and listen to what He has to say to us without interruption, as Matthew 14:23 reminds us:

> After He had dismissed the crowds, He went up on the mountain by Himself to pray. When it was evening, He was there alone.

When Jesus needed an answer from His Father, He turned to a place of solitude. Yet nowadays, it's hard to find time to be alone. The moment we realize that we're by ourselves, we reach for our phones or other forms of distraction. We even turn to these things when we're present with others, creating an unhealthy type of solitude that keeps us from getting to know them on a deeper level.

I've found that we avoid solitude because we're often afraid to face ourselves. We're scared that when we're left with nothing but our thoughts, we'll have to address things about ourselves or our lives that we may not be prepared to take on or recognize. But I have grown more spiritually from solitude than from perhaps any other aspect of my life. For it's in solitude that God often reveals where we may be struggling or what we may be in denial about.

The next time you find yourself alone, don't feel anxious—be elated instead. See that moment for what it really is . . . an uninterrupted few minutes to build not only your relationship with God but with yourself.

Offer

We learn how to have a healthier, deeper relationship with God when we fully embody the relationships we have here on earth. That's why what I propose today is the opposite of being alone, all in an effort to reveal how vital being alone with God truly is.

Today you'll devote the entire day to someone you care about deeply—the person you can be most yourself with. Give this person all your attention, which means no social media, incoming phone calls, or anything that detracts or distracts.

When we're in the company of (and focused solely on) someone we're close with, it can feel like a place of solitude, even though we're technically not alone. Just being able to be yourself—your true self— feels so easy and natural when there are no barriers around you and nothing between you and that person.

By day's end, not only will you end up with a stronger bond, but you'll be reminded of the greater level of intimacy that comes from being one-on-one with someone who loves you—and giving that person all of you. It reminds us that the same degree of closeness is reachable with God when we choose to devote time alone with Him—and no one else.

Sleep

Tonight, while lying in bed, try placing your fingertips on your wrist—or put your hand either over your heart or around your navel—and feel your heartbeat. Don't count or think about anything. All you should do is *feel* at that moment. Just concentrate on each beat as if it were a note in a song.

By carving out this time, you're giving yourself a few minutes of solitude that lets the rest of the world fall away. And if it doesn't, that's fine as well, because that's not necessarily what this is about. This act is more of a gesture that temporarily connects us to the life we're blessed to have. It's a reminder that our hearts are speaking to us every second of each day of our lives, just as God is speaking to us every second of each day as well. All it takes sometimes are a few seconds of silence so that you don't miss a beat of what He has to share with you.

Exercise

Today is an Acknowledge-Pray-Rest Day. Allow your body to recover from what you accomplished on Days 26 and 27 by forgoing any form of strength-training exercise. However, if you wish to walk with God on this day, you may do so as long as your Worship Walk doesn't exceed thirty minutes and you maintain a relaxed, comfortable pace. If you wish to spend additional time with Him, I encourage you to spend that time in prayer to allow your body to recover and heal.

Nutrition

On Day 25, I asked that you establish a food curfew, which in itself is a form of solitude. By setting a time limit, you're removing yourself from the potential temptation of eating foods you may not need to sustain yourself.

Today try considering individuals in your life who may tempt you to eat Faith-Less Foods or consume more food than you should. It can be difficult when those we love ask us to take a bite of an unhealthy dish they may be enjoying or prepare a meal for us that may not mesh with our own dietary goals. So ask yourself: Are the people around me during meal times lifting me toward my goals or making them harder for me to achieve?

Think about your surroundings and who you're with during moments when you are tempted to stray from Faith-Full Foods. If you feel your friends make things more challenging, then prepare yourself beforehand so that your get-togethers don't derail your journey. Eating something beforehand can help, as can simply insisting that you have an urge for something healthier at that moment.

The thing to keep in mind is this: Those who care about you will understand your choices, while those who take offense may not have your best interest at heart. They may even want you to succumb to poor eating habits so that they feel better about theirs. Stay strong in these moments, and recognize that the only person in the room who should decide what you eat is you.

DAY 29 (SUNDAY)

THE FIFTH SUNDAY

The Week of Glorification
(Days 29 through 35)

The purpose of Seven Sundays has always been, first and foremost, about strengthening your relationship with Him. With many things now in place regarding your sleep, exercise, and nutrition, it's time to build that bond further by stepping into your faith at an even higher level.

I believe that a lot of times when we're almost at the finish line, we let up a little bit. It's human nature to take it easy when we can see the end of our journey. But coming to God and thanking Him, praising Him, and worshipping Him in these times, it creates a different type of mind-set. It can give us a massive boost of energy that doesn't allow us to coast through but soar upward. That's why this week, you will glorify Him to help yourself grow even further.

Concede

Father, I make a declaration on this day to be thankful. There's nothing I want more than to enter into Your presence. I know that this declaration will push me deeper and break down walls that may be holding me back from revealing more of my heart to You. I praise You with thanksgiving because You are deserving of all the praise. Thank You, Father. Amen.

Honor

To start this week of glorification, I find inspiration in Psalm 100:4.

> *Enter His gates with a song of thanksgiving*
> *And His courts with praise.*
> *Be thankful to Him, bless and praise His name.*

The verse talks about celebrating and worshipping. But how often do you find yourself doing that? More often, I find that we tend to focus on what's difficult and how much work we may have ahead. Thinking about them can make ordinary tasks seem more arduous, invasive, or time-consuming than they really are. But when we let ourselves be thankful for the opportunities God has given us, when we are grateful for being busy, when we are appreciative that we have the means and health to take on these tasks, it makes the difficult things in life seem much more manageable.

So today be thankful—especially when things seem trying or tiring. Feel blessed for every opportunity, and question whether what appears unmanageable is only that way because that's how you perceive it to be.

Offer

Opening up your home is an offering unto itself. You're allowing people you trust to step into your personal space to share your environment in fellowship. You're bringing someone into a place that's your sanctuary of sorts.

Today extend an invitation to a few people to come over to where you live, either for breakfast before church, brunch afterward, or just to spend a few hours talking and enjoying each other's company. I know what you're thinking. Maybe the thought of having to clean up your house sounds like too much work, but that's actually not what I'm asking you to do. I don't want your concerns about how messy your house might be to interfere with the opportunity to connect with others. Instead remind yourself that you're not doing this to impress; you're doing it to enjoy the company of people—those you care enough about to welcome them into your life and who care about you. Trust that they won't mind any disorganization, just as you trust them to be in your home.

Sleep

With your sleep environment almost in synch, the only change you'll be making throughout this upcoming week will be reflecting on how you pray at night, particularly right before bedtime.

Every day from this point onward, I'll be suggesting tips for you to consider in order to experience prayer differently at night. That said, these will only be suggestions. I never want you to get too caught up in structure because when it comes to prayer, you should always be free. The way you pray should always be an individual experience. However, trying something new may allow you to draw more from prayer than may otherwise occur. Keep that in mind this week.

Exercise

Today is another Acknowledge-Pray-Rest Day. Allow your body to continue recovering from Days 26 and 27. You may walk with Him for up to thirty minutes at a relaxed, comfortable pace, but if you have been experiencing difficulty with the exercise portion of Seven Sundays, rest on this second day in a row away from exercise and spend that time in prayer instead.

Even if you're feeling strong and energized, you may want to use today to rest since the exercise portion this week is the most intense of the Seven Sundays program so far. However, know that it's nothing you cannot handle. In fact, keep that thought top of mind as you enter each workout. God teaches us that it's so important to take on challenges and persevere so that we may understand what we're each capable of. This week, try pushing past any discomfort and rejoice that you have such an opportunity to test yourself.

Nutrition

As a follower of Christ, you may already know about fasting as a spiritual discipline (denying oneself food, either completely or partially, for a certain amount of time). Throughout both the Old and New Testaments, there are many examples of fasting as a religious practice for a variety of reasons, such as when David fasted to show grief for the death of Abner or when the Israelites fasted to win back God's favor. Even Jesus fasted—for forty days!—in the desert.

Fasting is not only a way to humble oneself before God; it also shows your spiritual strength and dedication. It's a self-sacrifice meant to help increase your faith. That's why starting tomorrow—and over the course of this week—you'll be performing "intermittent fasting"; you'll be cycling between periods of not eating from 8:00 p.m. until noontime (12:00 p.m.) the following day, then eating four meals/snacks between noon and 8:00 p.m.

Beyond the spiritual growth you'll experience by glorifying God through intermittent fasting, your physical body will also benefit—and not simply from consuming fewer calories. Intermittent fasting (IF) *is* a form of weight control, since by reducing the amount of time you eat each day, you'll essentially be skipping meals. But depriving yourself of calories (and energy) triggers hormesis, a response to stress that causes your body to become more resilient. Because of that reaction, IF has also been shown to lower bad cholesterol (LDL), inflammation, blood glucose levels, and blood pressure, which can decrease your risk of heart disease, diabetes, cancer, and even aging.[1]

In order to get ready for this week, consider four things today:

Look at Your Health. There is a caveat to consider. If you are pregnant or lactating, diabetic, under age eighteen, or taking prescription drugs, or if you have any underlying medical problems, you should avoid this portion of Seven Sundays or check with a doctor to see if it's okay for you to try intermittent fasting.

Look in Your Fridge. Because you need to be ready to eat at a specific time, getting meals and snacks together beforehand will ensure that you'll stick to the schedule as planned, so think ahead.

Look at the Calendar. You may need to rethink any scheduled activities that might conflict with your fast, particularly at breakfast time or after 8:00 p.m. (two occasions when you won't be allowed to eat). If necessary, reschedule to avoid any potential get-togethers or meetings that might make it more difficult to abstain from eating.

Look in the Mirror Your first inclination might be to eat as much as possible today, knowing what you're about to undertake starting tomorrow. However, avoid that temptation and trust the process. Put your faith forward, instead of fearing what you'll soon be exploring.

DAY 30 (MONDAY)

Concede

Father, help me with my lack of faith because it's holding me back from my victories. I seek clarity as to why there's unbelief in me; give me understanding about why I feel this way so that I can begin to be bold in my faith. I yearn to share a deeper faith with You than I've ever had before. The victory I seek is not of the world, but a heavenly reward, one that's permanent and sustains my faith while I'm here on this earth. Thank You, Father. Amen.

Honor

Your relationship with God isn't founded on merit or on meeting certain conditions. It's based on faith and belief, which Hebrews 11:6 tells us must be in place if we wish to please God:

> *But without faith it is impossible to please Him, for whoever comes to God must believe that God exists and that He rewards those who seek Him.*

Fasting is one of the most powerful of all the spiritual disciplines we can offer as Christians. By humbling ourselves before God through fasting, we are seeking more clarity. We are asking Him to remove some of the distractions within our lives so that we may grow even closer to Him. We are showing God that our faith in Him is absolute and unchanging.

As you move through this day as well as this week, realize that this fast isn't about how much weight you may lose or how many healthier foods you may incorporate into your diet. It's about how much you believe in Him, trust in Him, and have faith in Him. That should always be your goal, as well as your guide.

Offer

If you've followed the Seven Sundays program faithfully, you'll have done so much for so many, in addition to making so many healthy changes for yourself. Even though every offering and lifestyle suggestion is rewarding in its own way, it's essential to truly reward yourself as well. That's why today's offering is all about you.

Today is about changing the way you talk to yourself—and treat yourself.

The way we respond to our mistakes dictates whether we'll make them again, along with how many others we may make down the road. Starting intermittent fasting today will most likely be entirely new to you, and if you've struggled with dietary changes in the past, it might feel like the hardest day of them all. But you need to know that you can do this because you're not the same person you were before Seven Sundays.

I also want to stress that Seven Sundays isn't a race, but a reinforcement of your relationship with God—and no relationship that's deep and meaningful is ever instant. If you think about the most significant relationships in your life, I'll bet you'll find that they took time and patience to build.

So give yourself some slack, and excuse yourself if you stumble starting today, just like you would forgive a friend, relative, or loved one. Don't expect perfection of yourself because the effort alone is what matters. You would never judge others for not being perfect, so why would you ever do the same to yourself?

Sleep

Today make the effort to pray before bedtime. If you already do so, then you're set. But if you typically don't, then from this day forward, try incorporating prayer before bedtime, in addition to whenever you usually pray throughout the day.

As I mentioned on Day 29, your prayer life is your own, so how you choose to do it—and how long you spend with Him—is entirely up to you. All I ask is that you pray—and just enjoy your time with Him.

This is important for two reasons. I'm a big believer in both starting and ending the day well. Nighttime prayer is an opportunity to grant ourselves a more peaceful sleep to help set the tone for the next day.

More important, it's a final opportunity for you to give thanks to God for His faithfulness throughout the day. It allows you to truly reflect on the many blessings He's given you that day that you may not have acknowledged at the moment. Through nighttime prayer, you can remember and relive them all.

Exercise

Today you'll walk outside with Him for twenty to thirty minutes, then do a mini-circuit of all five outdoor exercises back-to-back with no rest in between.

- Start by doing Push-ups for twenty repetitions.
- Next, you'll perform Lunges for twenty repetitions (each leg).

- Next, do the Moving Plank for sixty seconds.
- From there, you'll perform Burpees for twenty repetitions.
- Finally, you'll do Supermans for thirty repetitions.
- Rest by jogging (either in place or forward) for one minute, then repeat the circuit twice more for a total of three circuits.

As always, you can perform the circuit directly before or after your Worship Walk, or walk ten to fifteen minutes first, perform the circuit, then finish your workout with an additional ten to fifteen minutes of walking.

Nutrition

Today and each day moving forward, you'll skip breakfast, then reduce your eating period to eight hours per day. Within that time, you'll allow yourself only three meals and one snack (spaced roughly two to three hours apart) and stick with only Faith-Full Foods. After your final meal, you'll fast for sixteen hours—then repeat.

If you typically wake up at 7:00 or 8:00 a.m., your daily eating habits would break down in the following manner:

- Launch meal: 12:00 p.m.
- Second meal: 3:00 p.m.
- Snack: 5:00 p.m.
- Dinner: 7:00 p.m.
- Fast: 8:00 p.m. to 12:00 p.m.

However, we all operate under different schedules, so *you* decide when it's best for you to fast. So long as you're sticking to a 16:8 schedule (meaning, fasting for sixteen hours and eating only during the additional eight hours of the day), that's entirely fine. For example:

- If you start eating at 7:00 a.m., stop eating and start fasting at 3:00 p.m.
- If you start eating at 11:00 a.m., stop eating and start fasting at 7:00 p.m.
- If you start eating at 2:00 p.m., stop eating and start fasting at 10:00 p.m.
- If you start eating at 6:00 p.m., stop eating and start fasting at 2:00 a.m.

At its core, all I'm really asking you to do is skip breakfast and make lunch your first meal of the day. Then, eat as you normally would, but have your last meal before eight o'clock—and that's really it. But before you start, keep the following suggestions in mind:

What You Can Drink. It's crucial to stay hydrated while doing intermittent fasting, so drink water often throughout the day. You may also have black coffee and tea, but not too close to bedtime.

What You Might Hear or Feel. Will your stomach grumble? Probably. Will there be times (especially in the morning) when your mind is telling you that you need to eat? Most likely. But these instances are not anything to be concerned about. Remind yourself that this initial change comes with a few growing pains, but your body will adjust.

DAY 31 (TUESDAY)

Concede

Father, help me let go of control. The reality is, I want to be completely consumed by the Holy Spirit. I feel the empowering of the Holy Spirit, but my ego and pride constantly get in the way. Show me how to trust the spirit again so that I can operate fully in Your design. Thank You, Father. Amen.

Honor

Luke 12:12 is such a short verse with so much to show us:

> *"For the Holy Spirit will teach you in that very hour what you ought to say."*

With prayer, some people worry about saying the right things, remembering to mention everyone they love, or giving God enough of their time. We try to figure out what words we need to speak to Him. But in actuality, prayer is a connection of the heart. It's not necessary to think about what you're saying if you allow the Holy Spirit to guide you.

That trust in the Holy Spirit applies not only to prayer, but to this journey—and throughout the rest of your life.

Sometimes what prevents us from moving forward is that we simply get in our own way. We feel the need to always be in control and have every answer. But what we may be doing in certain situations is blocking the Holy Spirit from speaking.

When we give a moment over to God and allow the Holy Spirit to come in and work through us, we're able to harness strength and find direction from it. But, most important, we are comforted by knowing that we don't always have to have all the answers to find happiness.

Offer

Today I'd like you to try looking for someone who seems down or distant and allowing the Holy Spirit to flow through you. When you open yourself to this idea before your day starts, you'll be surprised by the number of people you'll see in need—and you'll be excited to have so many opportunities to make someone feel good this day.

If you personally know of someone who could use some cheering up, you can write a kind e-mail, send a card, or place flowers on their desk or doorstep. But I don't want you to have too many boundaries on this day.

The experience can be brief and doesn't even have to be deeply personal. Paying a compliment, being positive, or doing something nice for someone can all lift someone else's spirit, and it only takes a few seconds. Even simply saying "Good morning!" or "Have a great day" may not feel like much, but if you're sincere, it might make someone feel a little better about their day.

Sleep

Today and throughout this week, I'll suggest a few things that I like to use when I pray at night. If any don't feel natural to you, you're free to step away from any or all of them. But I find that when I incorporate certain things into my nightly prayer, I get much more from those moments alone with Him as a result.

The first suggestion ties directly into the theme for this day, which is to step away from your usual prayer and allow yourself to be led by the Holy Spirit. Shy away from your usual conversation with Him by starting in silence and allowing the Holy Spirit to shape your thoughts and words. Don't worry about things you forget to mention or if you spend less time than usual with God. Let whatever comes forth come forth tonight, and know that whatever is revealed was meant to be revealed.

Exercise

Today you'll move through a circuit of all five indoor exercises back-to-back with no rest in between.

- Start by performing the Double-Pump Shoulder Press for twenty repetitions.
- From there, you'll perform Dips for twenty repetitions.
- Next, you will do Squat & Holds for twenty repetitions.
- After that, you will do Step Ups for twenty repetitions (each leg).
- Finally, you'll get on the ground and do Bicycles for thirty repetitions.
- Rest for one minute by walking (or standing) in place, then repeat the mini-circuit twice more for a total of three circuits.

Nutrition

Today you'll continue to fast for sixteen hours off and eight hours on. But to make things easier, I encourage you to create a few distractions that are not based on food to fill your mornings this week.

Not having anything to do immediately upon waking can make you more eager to reach for food out of boredom or force of habit. If on this morning or any of your mornings this week, it seems that you may not have enough activity to distract you until noon, consider arranging your schedule in a way that keeps you more active in the morning.

DAY 32 (WEDNESDAY)

Concede

Secure me, Father, in all this chaos. The world around me is constantly changing, and there seems to be so much confusion. I want to show that no matter what's going on in the world, You are my savior. As long as I stay connected to You, I have hope. Thank You, Father. Amen.

Honor

Our circumstances are constantly changing; our career, relationships, interests—they all change. We change too, sometimes through effort and determination, and sometimes without our consent. But there's one thing that always remains steadfast, as Hebrews 13:8 reminds us:

> *Jesus Christ is the same yesterday and today and forever.*

We should be reassured knowing that He remains the same, no matter how much our lives change. He is the same today as He was yesterday and will be tomorrow. No matter what, He always loves us, and He will never leave us or forsake us.

That lesson is so important, particularly during days when change may feel overwhelming. You should feel a sense of peace and security knowing that no matter what changes around you, good or bad, God's love will remain constant.

Offer

What is unchanging is how God is always there for us, and He always keeps His promises. We should keep ours as well.

This may seem like an easy offering, but not all of us live up to our word at every turn. We may say we're going to do something but quickly forget, reschedule, or pass because life gets busy. Sometimes we may even break a promise if something better comes up. That's why I hope from this day forward that if you make a promise—if you commit to doing something for someone—you'll make that obligation a priority.

Sometimes that will mean turning down another opportunity that comes along. In that case, you'll have to trust God and know that there will be other opportunities.

When we're true to our word, it shows character and exemplifies what it means to be a Christian. It also creates stronger relationships with others, as they come to understand that we're genuinely there for them when they need us. You will become recognized as someone they can put more faith into.

I also think it's important to be bold with our promises, so go out on a limb for someone whom you normally wouldn't put yourself out there for. Often it's easier to keep promises to people closest to us, but easier to dismiss them with those who are outside of our lives. Make sure to keep these promises, as they show the most commitment.

Sleep

As you continue to pray each evening, ask God to help you rest so you'll be better prepared for tomorrow. Bringing my sleep into my prayer gives me a sense of peace that I can't quite explain, but when you try it, you'll see what I mean. It's comforting to know that He is looking after me and protecting me as I sleep.

Praying for good rest also acts as a reminder that we can ask for His heavenly hand for all kinds of things that are important in our lives. He is always there for us, whether we need help having better judgment, patience, focus, confidence, or anything else.

Exercise

Today is an Acknowledge-Pray-Rest Day. Allow your body to recover from what you accomplished on Days 30 and 31 by forgoing any form of strength-training exercise. However, if you wish to walk with God today, you may do so as long as your Worship Walk doesn't exceed thirty minutes, and you maintain a relaxed, comfortable pace. If you wish to spend additional time with Him, I encourage you to spend that time in prayer to allow your body to recover and heal.

Nutrition

You're three days into your fast, and by now, you've most likely encountered a few social situations that may have left you seeking solutions. If you found yourself in a setting where fasting was either difficult or you felt uncomfortable, here are a few strategies you can use next time:

- Just explain that you're not hungry or that you're saving your appetite for lunch (if it's morning). If it's after 8:00 p.m., just say you had a big dinner, and no one should question why you're not eating.
- If that's not possible and you still feel self-conscious about not having something in your hand, ask for a glass of water or a cup of plain coffee or tea instead.

- Final option: Just own it! This journey may be about strengthening your relationship with God, but along the way, whether you realize it or not, you are serving as an example to others. By explaining what you're doing and why you're doing it, you may encourage the people around you to try this journey for themselves.

The important thing is to not make people feel like you don't want to spend time with them just because you're not eating. Being open about your journey will allow you to let people around you know you're there for *them*—and not necessarily for the meal you would've eaten.

DAY 33 (THURSDAY)

Concede

Father, this is my favorite part of the day. I love spending time with You. I love how You show me new things. You constantly surprise me. I want to continue this journey with You, but I often get caught up doing things that distract me from this time with You. I surrender to Your Word and Your Spirit, as this is the most critical thing in my life. Thank You, Father. Amen.

Honor

The Word of God isn't simply something to read and remember, but something that needs to be ruminated on, as Psalm 119:15–16 reminds us:

> I will meditate on Your precepts
> And regard Your ways.
> I will delight in Your statutes;
> I will not forget Your word.

Sometimes we overlook the meaning of Scripture when we simply read it. But contemplating the Word of God helps us understand on a more profound level just how practical its meaning is—and how it connects seamlessly into our own lives. Instead of just reading verses, repeat them in your mind and visualize their meaning. Let His message sink into your spirit and become a part of you.

When that happens, the Word of God changes how we operate. It gives us insight that we otherwise may never be granted. I've watched it transform my own prayer life in a way that has immeasurably strengthened my relationship with God. Now prayer feels as if I am talking to a good friend, and that effect makes me eagerly seek out more time with Him throughout the day.

Offer

When there's chaos in our lives, we always have two choices. We can be swept up by the disarray and become part of it. Or we can remain calm and try to play a part in solving it. Today (and moving forward), there will only be one option to pick from: you'll always be the cooler head that prevails, especially during times when you normally wouldn't remain composed.

Staying calm sets the tone in every area of your life. When we lose our temper or patience, we are saying that we have lost partial control of ourselves. That alone can make it much harder for others to be as receptive to whatever it is we need to say.

When we embody a sense of calm, everyone around us feels respected and heard. It also minimizes the chance that we might say or do things we may regret later on. But, perhaps most important, handling a situation with grace also rubs off on others and makes them aspire to find that patience within themselves. Even if someone else isn't being calm at that moment, your sense of calm forces that person to step back from their actions. You end up leading by example—showing others how to let go of panic and frustration, and instead replace them with courtesy and reason.

Sleep

One thing I like to do during nighttime prayer is to reflect back on scripture that I've read in the morning to see how my understanding of that scripture has changed through the course of the day.

By coming back to a specific passage at the end of the day, you may notice something you missed in the morning, or you might appreciate it in another way. It can be like admiring a piece of art at different times of the day or from various angles. It's the same masterpiece, but when you come back to it, you may see details that would have otherwise gone unnoticed.

Since you're already reflecting upon each day's Honoring throughout the day as part of Seven Sundays, you can always add it into your nighttime prayer and ask yourself: Do I see something in this passage that I hadn't seen before? Or if you wish, feel free to choose other passages to explore from morning until night.

Exercise

Today you'll walk outside with Him for twenty to thirty minutes, then do a mini-circuit of all five outdoor exercises back-to-back with no rest in between.

- Start by doing Push-ups for twenty repetitions.
- Next, you'll perform Lunges for twenty repetitions (each leg).
- Next, do the Moving Plank for sixty seconds.
- From there, you'll perform Burpees for twenty repetitions.
- Finally, you'll do Supermans for thirty repetitions.
- Rest by jogging (either in place or forward) for one minute, then repeat the circuit twice more for a total of three circuits.

Nutrition

I'm confident that in the four days you've been realigning yourself with God through fasting, you've experienced hunger pangs and cravings—and that's normal. However, that doesn't mean that you don't have power over these feelings. Being wise during the times you're allowed to eat can ease some of that discomfort—if you choose the right type of foods. Some ideas that may help you stay on the path include:

Consider Eating Even More Fiber-rich Foods.

If you haven't been incorporating very many Faith-Full Foods from Days 11 and 12, now is the time to double down on eating vegetables, oatmeal, and other high-fiber foods. They keep you feeling full longer.

Even if You Think You're Drinking Enough Water, You Probably Aren't.

Keep a glass right by your bed, and make drinking it the first thing you do when you get up. Then keep drinking as often as possible throughout the day until a few hours before bedtime (you'll want to stop then so it doesn't affect your sleep).

Eating Slow-digesting Food as Part of Your Last Meal of the Day Can Help Curb Hunger before You Sleep.

Look for foods that contain casein protein (the type of protein found in milk products, which takes about six to eight hours for your body to digest) or healthy fats (which also take roughly eight hours to digest). A few suggestions to possibly mix into your final meal of the day could include:

- A serving of cottage cheese and a handful of almonds
- A serving of Greek yogurt with a teaspoon of Chia seeds
- A scoop of casein protein powder (you can find it at any supermarket, drugstore, or health food store) and a tablespoon of organic peanut butter

(By the way: There are a lot of different casein protein powders out there on the market, which can make it difficult to choose. One way to make sure you pick the best option is to identify powders that don't have any additives, such as artificial flavorings, colors, or sweeteners. Though these all-natural powders are the healthier options, you may find their flavor a little bland. To sweeten things up, I recommend adding between one-half and a full serving of stevia to taste. Just mix a scoop of powder with a few ounces of water and shake well; that's all you need.)

DAY 34 (FRIDAY)

Concede

Father, I know that there is creativity within me. I'm not asking You to give me more of it, but to help me embrace the creativity that You have already blessed me with, so that I can unleash and truly become the person You have created me to be. Make it clear to me how I can use my creativity to bless the world. Thank You, Father. Amen.

Honor

1 Timothy 4:14–15 speaks about the gifts we are given—and how we should always both appreciate and nurture them:

> *Do not neglect the spiritual gift within you, which was intentionally bestowed on you through prophetic utterance when the elders laid their hands on you. Practice and work hard on these things; be absorbed in them, so that your progress will be evident to all.*

Even though we're all unique and have our own variety of abilities, skill sets, and gifts, I believe we all share certain traits—and one of them is creativity.

One of the biggest misconceptions is that creativity can only be expressed in artistic areas such as painting, writing, or music. But we're all imaginative in our own way, and creativity can find its way into anything. If, for you, that means thinking of a new way to organize your daily schedule or ways to rearrange furniture, that is a creative pursuit. The important thing is to keep in mind that there is no right or wrong way to express creativity, so let it shine without fear of failure.

If you don't recognize where your creativity lies, try challenging yourself to think about things in your life in a more creative way. Think about something that could be implemented at work that's never been done before, or what you might do with an empty space on your wall. Invent a fun activity to do with your children, or just doodle on a piece of paper each day.

Your creativity is always there for you, and coaxing it out sometimes just means letting yourself feel free enough to allow all things that come to your mind to flow out.

Offer

This day isn't only about embracing your creativity; it's also about encouraging and supporting other people's creative spirit. The beauty of knowing everyone has creativity within themselves is that you know there are always creative people around you. So today, when you see examples of others' creativity, compliment them and ask them a little bit more about what they have brought to life.

Recognizing a person's creativity builds confidence within that person, and they keep going out on a limb to let their originality flow. You inspire them to tap into their creative muscle more and more. Whether it's a picture someone drew, the way they dress or arrange their house, the ideas they come up with, or the way they organize themselves, praise their ingenuity and ask what inspired it.

Even if you don't understand someone's creative viewpoint, try to support their enthusiasm. Sometimes creativity needs a little push in the form of a pat on the back. The person you're complimenting might be stalled creatively and may just need a glimmer of support to feel confident enough to move on.

The truth is, creativity is never-ending, and it often takes time. For some, it may require days of effort, while for others, it might take decades to express what's in their heart, mind, and spirit. Each person you meet may be in a place where they need to hear a few heartening words to move forward. By just saying "I love how creative you are! How did you think of that?" you may indirectly keep someone's creativity ignited so that they might dream up even more glorious ideas or creations that may inspire others.

Sleep

As I get ready for bed, I like to go back through my day in my mind and repent for the sins I may have committed that day. I find that accounting and atoning for my actions each day has a definite impact.

I don't simply repent for things that I've done that day, but I also try to look beyond the physical. I'll address specific emotions that may have crept into my heart, such as fear, jealousy, or doubt. I'll look at feelings or thoughts I had that day that didn't make me proud and that I need to work on.

When I address these things with God head-on, it forces me to admit and apologize for my mistakes in a way that makes me less likely to make those choices again or have those thoughts the next day. But repenting also allows me to clear those sins away before I rest. By not shying away from what God already knows and admitting my sins to Him each evening, I gain a sense of ease. I'm reminded that I am a work in progress and that He loves me anyway.

Exercise

On this day, you'll move through a circuit of all five indoor exercises back-to-back with no rest in between.

- Start by performing the Double-Pump Shoulder Press for twenty repetitions.
- From there, you'll perform Dips for twenty repetitions.
- Next, you will do Squat & Holds for twenty repetitions.
- After that, you will do Step Ups for twenty repetitions (each leg).
- Finally, you'll get on the ground and do Bicycles for thirty repetitions.
- Rest for one minute by walking (or standing) in place, then repeat the mini-circuit twice more for a total of three circuits.

Nutrition

You should have begun to see a turn in how your body deals with fasting. Your body has finally adjusted and is starting to utilize its resources in a way it wasn't before this process. It should now be working for you instead of against you.

When you eat all day long, your body is constantly burning off food and doesn't get an opportunity to utilize stored fat. Even though everyone's metabolism is a little different, your body should now be used to tapping into its fat stores more often.

———

Everyone's body works differently, but by improving how you eat, sleep, and exercise, your actions until now should have made this experience less of a struggle than it would be if you hadn't already made those changes. But if you still feel like you're struggling, then keep this in mind: When I feel that slight discomfort, it fuels me to push myself a little bit further. It's a physical reminder that I'm temporarily stepping away from something to help me develop a closer walk with Him. It's also when I find Matthew 6:16 a source of motivation:

> *"And whenever you are fasting, do not look gloomy like the hyp-ocrites, for they put on a sad and dismal face so that their fasting may be seen by men. I assure you and most solemnly say to you, they have their reward in full."*

There are layers of meaning here, but for now I want to point out this: Fasting isn't meant to be completely comfortable, but we aren't supposed to focus on it and draw attention to it. The temporary discomfort you may be experiencing is merely something that many other Christians have gone through as well.

Remember: This journey is *your* important religious event, and what you're doing is a token of deep and sincere dedication to Him. So do not look gloomy, and instead feel glorious.

DAY 35 (SATURDAY)

Concede

Father, I want my entire self to be a living sacrifice to You. I want to worship You with my mind, body, and spirit. Forget about all the ritual traditions and laws; teach me real worship. I ask that You reveal to me things that I may be putting ahead of You. My focus is to put You at the forefront of my life by surrendering all distractions over to You. Thank You, Father. Amen.

Honor

Today, reflect upon Romans 12:1:

> *Therefore I urge you, brothers and sisters, by the mercies of God, to present your bodies as a living sacrifice, holy and well-pleasing to God, which is your rational act of worship.*

Surrendering to God's plan for us may mean sacrificing our comfort or our conveniences, but think about what he's sacrificed for us. Jesus himself sacrificed glory, position, and even the acceptance of others to walk with us before giving His life for us.

As you prepare to embark on the final week of Seven Sundays—the week of dedication—remember the importance of being a living, walking sacrifice for God. Let everything that you do from this point forward be for His benefit as you put the Lord first above self. Do what He has called you to do and give your body over to righteousness, and let every act of your body be an act of worship. Make every action an example to others that Christ is more precious to you than anything else.

Offer

Many of us sacrifice portions of ourselves all day long, often without realizing it. We may sacrifice our time or energy to do things that do not serve Him. We may sacrifice our happiness or beliefs in order to please. We may sacrifice our privacy or dignity to gain attention or feel connected.

Even though you're to be a walking sacrifice for Him, that doesn't mean you should be sacrificing certain things about yourself along the way. So today look for the obstacles in your life that are leading to any unhealthy forms of sacrifice. By that I mean sacrifices that aren't bringing you closer to Him.

I'm not talking about the sacrifices we make for people we love, because relationships are all about compromise. Being a good parent, spouse, partner, or sibling is a delicate balance, one that often requires a sacrifice of your own needs. I'm referring to the sacrifices you shouldn't be making, which are sacrifices that may be affecting the following:

Your health
Your self-worth
Your integrity
Your personal safety
Your identity
Your spiritual needs

If you're making any sacrifices right now that are diminishing any of these aspects of your life, reconsider your actions in these instances—and step away from any situations that are causing you to sacrifice unnecessarily.

Sleep

If you've ever given a speech, you already know the importance of reading it aloud beforehand. Reading it aloud helps us notice things we might otherwise not detect if we're just reading to ourselves. Hearing the words aloud causes us to reflect on their impact and helps us determine if what we're trying to say is making the point we're hoping to make. That's why tonight I encourage you to pray aloud.

Don't whisper or merely mouth the words. Instead speak with God as if He is right there in front of you—because He is.

Talking directly to God puts us more in tune with the message we want to convey to Him and gives each word more authority. Also, the more we vocalize what you're trying to share with Him, the more likely you'll think about other things you wish to say as well. Speaking aloud can broaden the conversation in a more productive way that you otherwise may never experience by keeping your prayers as thoughts.

Exercise

Today is an Acknowledge-Pray-Rest Day, and after such a hard week of exercise, enjoy this day, because you've earned it. Allow your body to recover from what you accomplished on Days 33 and 34 by forgoing any form of strength-training exercise. However, if you wish to walk with God on this day, you may do so as long as your Worship Walk doesn't exceed thirty minutes and you maintain a relaxed, comfortable pace. If you wish to spend additional time with Him, I encourage you to spend that time in prayer to allow your body to recover and heal.

Nutrition

Over the course of next week, you'll continue with a modified version of intermittent fasting, but you'll focus on the types of foods mentioned in Daniel 1:12–15.

> *"Please, test your servants for ten days, and let us be given some vegetables to eat and water to drink. Then let our appearance and the appearance of the young men who eat the king's finest food be observed and compared by you, and deal with your servants in accordance with what you see." So the man listened to them in this matter and tested them for ten days. At the end of ten days it seemed that they were looking better and healthier than all the young men who ate the king's finest food.*

The gist of the story is that Daniel and his men abstained from food declared unclean by God in the Laws of Moses for ten days. During that length of time, they abstained from meat, leavened and sweet bread, and wine. Instead they only ate vegetables—in some translations, "pulses,"—which are "foods grown from seed." And at the end of those ten days, they were better in appearance and fatter in flesh (which meant "stronger" in that time).

Not only was there a physical transformation, but God had blessed Daniel and those who fasted with him with many things, including favor, learning, and skill, as well as literature and wisdom, and understanding in all visions or dreams.

Today and throughout the rest of your journey, you'll be sticking to the same rules you've been following over the previous week. I still want you to fast for sixteen hours a day and eat only during eight hours a day, eating at least three meals within that eight-hour window. The only difference is that you'll only be eating certain types of Faith-Full Foods, including:

All fruits (fresh, frozen, juiced, but not canned. Dried is also acceptable if nothing man-made is added)

All whole grains (such as oats, millet, quinoa, barley, and brown rice)

All vegetables

All nuts and seeds

All beans and legumes (fresh is preferred, although canned is acceptable as long as there is no additional salt or other additives)

Water

This kind of diet is sometimes referred to as the Daniel Fast, since it's drawn from the story of Daniel. There are whole books about this topic, but I've studied the verses in the Bible and given you my own version of the plan outlined in Scripture. If you doubt your ability to stick with this diet, know that you've already built a solid foundation over this last week. The only change you're making is the foods you're eating—and for a good reason. This final step is about bringing you to a place where you haven't been with God before. It's about taking that last leap by making this temporary sacrifice one that will assuredly bring you closer to Him.

DAY 36 (SUNDAY)

THE SIXTH SUNDAY

The Week of Dedication
(Days 36 through 42)

This is it—the final stretch of Seven Sundays, and what may be for you the most rewarding week of all. In some ways, these last days will be more comfortable than last week, but they will be trying in others. When it gets tough, know that everything you've accomplished until now has prepared you for this seven-day test of devotion.

Concede

Father, how can I abide in You more? I don't want my love to be mere words, but I want to show You through my actions how much You mean to me. I want it to be my affection that drives me closer to You. I want to obey You out of love and not from my own strength. Thank You, Father. Amen.

Honor

One of my favorite passages is John 14:23:

> *Jesus answered, "If anyone loves Me, he will keep My word; and My Father will love him, and We will come to him and make Our dwelling place with him."*

Sometimes we get too caught up in the *doing* part of showing obedience to God. When we simply open our hearts even further to Him, love becomes the cause of our obedience. Love drives us to obey Him and guides our actions, instead of feeling that if we do certain things, we will receive good things from Him.

When we fast, we're trying to galvanize our relationship with God and bring it to another level through an act of obedience. It's about clearing away things so that we may hear God's voice a little better and know what His path is for us.

Even though this journey has asked you to do many things, you aren't required you do a single one. What you take on has always been up to you, just as performing actions throughout this final week are up to you as well. All I ask is that you open your heart as wide as you can, and I think you'll find that what may seem challenging may be something you cherish upon completion, especially when you realize that what kept you strong throughout was His love—and your love for Him.

Offer

Just lending an ear and being a sounding board is not only a powerful way to connect with someone, but a terrific exercise in remaining selfless. Today you'll reveal your heart by opening your ears and showing respect by genuinely listening to everyone you come in contact with.

Most of us believe ourselves to be great listeners, but often we are merely listening for an opportunity to switch the conversation back to ourselves. We may hear about someone else's achievements or issues, then immediately reflect our own back toward that person.

I can always tell when someone isn't really listening to me with all their heart, and I imagine you can as well. When we sense that distance, it makes us hold ourselves back from being as vulnerable with them. Others can sense the same thing in us. It keeps them from opening up as much and connecting with us. By not being as attentive, not only do we miss the chance to bond with that individual, but we may ignore the fact that we may not get as many opportunities in the future.

Today try not to bat conversations back and forth like a tennis match. Instead, try focusing entirely on what each person has to say; let the only things coming from your mouth be questions that relate to what they've already said. That way, they may speak more about themselves and whatever they're going through or proud of at that moment.

How you listen is just as important as listening itself. Before the other person speaks, try to minimize any distractions (putting your phone away, and maybe suggesting a quieter place to speak). As they talk, focus your eyes on them (not others around you) and face your body toward them. Don't cross your arms if you can help it.

I'm not asking you to be speechless. You may give advice, but only if counsel is asked for. Exercise patience and try to avoid thinking about what you're going to say next. Instead just listen to the words—every single word—and keep the conversation aimed at the other person.

Sleep

During this final week, you'll begin to turn off all electronics a minimum of ten to fifteen minutes before bedtime, so that by next Sunday you'll be "fasting" from electronics for up to ninety minutes before bedtime. Today I want you to be yourself, but be aware of what time you finally stop using anything electronic for the day.

For most of us, that tends to be right before bedtime. This affects us both physically and spiritually. The bright glow of a screen—even from the tiniest sources, such as a cell phone or tablet—can signal your brain to stay awake by stimulating photoreceptors within the retinas of our eyes that sense light and dark. The light from devices is also short-wavelength-enriched and has a higher concentration of what is known as "blue light," a type of light known to suppress levels of the sleep-inducing hormone melatonin. The more blue light you're exposed to prior to bedtime, the greater your risk of taking longer to fall asleep and experiencing less REM sleep, so you end up feeling sleepier than you should upon waking up.

You can set your phone or install an app that changes the colors on your screen, reducing blue light to warmer colors, such as reds and yellows. I encourage you to do this so you're looking at a warmer screen a few hours before bedtime. But minimizing screen time this week goes beyond just changing the light. We're going to look at changing your habits to improve your sleep and general well-being. The reason is this: Constantly "checking in" with work, your favorite show, or the Internet usually means you are "checking out" when it comes to spending quality time with Him, your family, your friends, and the things that truly matter in life. For most of us, the evening hours are the most precious because that's when we tend to be around those we love. By minimizing the hold electronics have on us, we can spend more time with the people who matter.

You may have a job or role that requires being "tuned in"—even during the final hours before sleep. If that's you, then just do your best to reprioritize a few things. It might be letting friends, family, and coworkers know that you're unavailable after a certain time this week. Or it may be doing things earlier in the day that you typically do at night. Whatever the case may be, consider reorganizing things or informing others so that this week's electronics fast will not interfere with other priorities.

Exercise

You're into the final stretch, and the good news is that the hardest workouts are now behind you. Because you're currently following a stricter intermittent fast, you'll be dialing back the intensity of your workouts.

This week you'll be performing the same routine as Week Three—the Week of Purification. However, if even this proves to be too intense for you, try dialing back the intensity even further. If what's recommended this week feels comfortable, or even too easy, then don't increase the intensity beyond what's recommended.

Nutrition

This last week is by far the most demanding nutritionally, but I also feel it's the most rewarding. It's a culmination of everything you've been working toward within each Pillar of Promise. That's why starting Monday, I'll be reminding you each day how you've gotten to this point of Seven Sundays.

There is nothing to prepare for, with the exception of the few Faith-Full Foods you may need to have on hand.

Instead, as you spend time in fellowship, take a moment to look around your church and consider what you're doing in His name. Draw strength from those worshipping alongside you and remind yourself that everyone around you is seeking that same closeness with Him. Connect to how your body feels so that you associate any slight hunger or mild discomfort as an affirmation of your commitment to God. Unite what you feel physically with where you are spiritually so that when your body speaks to you throughout this week, your spirit will fall back to this peaceful and positive moment in His house.

DAY 37 (MONDAY)

Concede

It's the last week, Father, and I need You to help me see this journey all the way through to the end. You say that if we wait on You, Lord, that You will renew our strength, that we will not grow weary but will soar on wings like eagles. I know that You contain everything I need, so I'm letting go and letting You lift me through this day. Thank You, Father. Amen.

Honor

Isaiah 40:31 is one of my favorite Scriptures to turn to:

> *But those who wait for the Lord*
> *Will gain new strength and renew their power;*
> *They will lift up their wings like eagles;*
> *They will run and not become weary,*
> *They will walk and not grow tired.*

This verse in particular speaks about "waiting" for Him. This is a message that's so important to keep top of mind, especially as you continue with this particular form of fasting.

When we wait for Him—meaning, when we anticipate and seek Him out—we're brought closer to God. He gives us strength when we need it most. When we wait for God, He is there to pick us up, to help us soar, and He fills us with energy everlasting. Remember that He is there to renew us—all it takes to make that happen is to place your hope in Him.

Offer

In our rush to move forward, we often fail to appreciate the importance of patience. We live in a world where speed and convenience are prized, but when you really look at the things that are meant to save us time, they're usually not healthier or better for us. For example, a text may be a faster way to communicate with someone, but it doesn't compare to speaking to that person. A frozen meal might take only minutes to prepare, but it doesn't compare to healthier home-cooked food.

That's why today try forgoing instant gratification in every endeavor, and instead do not just *wait*, but appreciate what waiting can offer you. Waiting shows our command of a situation and helps us learn how to use our energy wisely instead of wastefully. It also teaches us empathy, tolerance, and humility. Perhaps most important, it helps us reprioritize what's really important. Often many of us are in a rush to go somewhere that is not necessarily important. We've just become accustomed to being first or getting what we want when we want it.

So today make yourself wait a few moments longer at every opportunity. Let someone in front of you while waiting in line, allow someone else to pull ahead of you while in traffic, make a meal that might take a little longer to prepare, or be early to an appointment, but don't reach for your phone to entertain yourself. Instead use the time you wait to allow the Holy Spirit to move through you. For it's in those moments when we take a little extra time to be patient that we recognize how lucky we are to have that time.

Sleep

Throughout this week, you'll begin to fast from all electronics (cell phone, TV, computer, tablet, and any other mechanical distractions). Today all I ask is that you turn everything off ten to fifteen minutes before bedtime. That means not taking any electronics to bed, so if you use your cell phone as an alarm clock, either raise its volume and place it in another room (so that you're not tempted to reach for it) or find another option to wake you up in the morning.

If this is the first time you've ever stepped away from technology before bedtime, you may find yourself a bit lost. That's great. I explained yesterday that technology before bedtime has become a root cause of sleeplessness, but it also tends to pull us away from developing deeper relationships with God and those closest to us.

Even though we may feel "connected" to others as we surf the web or sift through e-mails or social media, the reality is that we're missing out on real opportunities to unite. We're missing out on moments that could be the best part of our entire day.

As you pull back on your technology use, you'll be replacing it with something that brings you even more in touch with God, with yourself, and those you love. Tonight you'll use the extra time gained to extend your nighttime prayer.

Often—whether we realize it or not—we tend to speak with God for a specific amount of time. We unconsciously put a time limit on something that should never have limitations. By adding this time to your prayer this evening, you'll notice something that you may never have given yourself the opportunity to experience. A more fruitful, fuller discussion that can only be had by giving God the extra time He deserves.

Exercise

Today you'll walk outside with Him for twenty to thirty minutes, then do a mini-circuit of all five outdoor exercises back-to-back with no rest in between.

- Start by doing Push-ups for twelve repetitions.
- Next, you'll perform Lunges for twelve repetitions (each leg).
- Next, do the Moving Plank for thirty seconds.
- From there, you'll perform Burpees for twelve repetitions.
- Finally, you'll do Supermans for twenty repetitions.
- Rest by jogging (either in place or forward) for one minute, then repeat the circuit once more for a total of two circuits.

If you're worried that you're not moving forward because this week isn't as intense as the last, fear not. The thing to remember is that when it comes to exercise, you don't always need to do more. If you never take the time to dial back your routine, it can not only lead to a mental and physical burnout but also increase your risk of injury. That's why it's imperative to lower the intensity of your workouts every six to eight weeks to give your body a full week's rest.

Bringing down the intensity while still going through the motions gives your body and spirit a breather without sacrificing results. In fact, you'll find that when you return to exercise soon after, you'll be more engaged and feel energized and physically refreshed.

Nutrition

As you stick to your fast of only eating at least three meals within an eight-hour window—choosing only certain types of Faith-Full Foods, which include fruits, whole grains, vegetables, nuts and seeds, beans, legumes, and water—consider this: Your first week of Seven

Sundays was about illumination, and one of the purposes of fasting is to get transparency about ourselves. It's a time for God to shine light into our lives so that we may understand more of our strengths and uncover the weaknesses that have been holding us back.

In John 8:12, it is said:

Once more Jesus addressed the crowd. He said, "I am the Light of the world. He who follows Me will not walk in the darkness, but will have the Light of life."

This scripture is really about allowing God to be the source that reveals things within us. So on this third day of your fast, remind yourself that God is the ultimate illuminator and that this is not a process you can do without Him.

I want you also to consider that the illumination that comes from fasting is never something we have to force. Often God will surprise us as we fast by showing us things that we've never noticed about ourselves, as well as about people and things within our own lives. It's okay to stay aware, but don't try to predict or anticipate what He will show you. Let God reveal what you need to know during this time when it is best for Him.

DAY 38 (TUESDAY)

Concede

Father, it's so easy for me to give, but so hard for me to receive. Why is it so difficult for me to trust and be vulnerable and to let love in? I want to let You in and allow You to be the healer of my soul. Come in and start shining Your light on me. I want to experience love in a whole new way. Thank You, Father. Amen.

Honor

In order to give love, you have to be full of love, and He is there to fill that space within each of us. But in order to allow God's love in, we need to understand how much He loves us, and there's no better scripture that explains the significance of God's love toward humanity than John 3:16:

> For God so loved and dearly prized the world, that He gave His only begotten Son, so that whoever believes and trusts in Him shall not perish, but have eternal life.

It means a lot when someone tells us that they love us. So you can only imagine that when God says He loves us, how immense that love must be. But sometimes it's easy to forget just how strong His love is for us.

However, when we give ourselves time to meditate on this scripture—when we remember how much He sacrificed for us, even though we didn't deserve it—we have the greatest example of His devotion for us. It allows us to see that through Him, we are already full of His love. All it takes is letting Him into your heart to receive His love. Once you do that, you'll have even more love to give to Him, everyone around you, and yourself.

Offer

Who do you love, and when was the last time you told them about it? More important, when you said, "I love you," do you think they knew how much you meant it?

Telling someone you love them only takes a second, but it's an action that can be difficult for many. It can leave some feeling vulnerable, while others may wonder why they have to declare their love when they show it in other ways.

Even when it's easy for us, we may throw out "I love you" with little regard or in a way that makes it carry less weight. But it's an expression that should never be spoken without feeling or merely used to close a conversation. Using the words lightly reduces their effectiveness and minimizes how you genuinely feel.

So today tell someone that you love them at a moment when they least expect to hear it. Try bringing it up in the middle of a conversation—or even at the beginning—instead of at the end. Call or reach out to someone specifically not just to check in with them, but to just tell them you love them. And when possible, always look them in the eyes and smile.

You may throw that person off guard or hear the words repeated back. Either way, it's okay, because this isn't about receiving—it's about giving. This moment is to let others know how you feel for them, with no expectation of having them be honest or as comfortable expressing what they feel for you.

Sleep

Tonight you'll continue with your electronic fast by turning off all electronics a minimum of twenty to thirty minutes before bedtime. To fill that void, consider listening to worship music in its place.

When we rely on electronics before bedtime, we often find ourselves completely disconnected from what's happening around us. Our electronic devices can place us in a different mind-set, but that mentality is typically never in tune with His message and what He wants for us.

Listening to worship music (or a sermon, if you so choose) is an expression that shows Him our gratitude and love. In its own way, it's a way of thanking Him for all the things He gives us. But, even more important, when we take the time to listen to music that glorifies Him and all the things He does for us, it puts us in a better state of mind and makes us feel grateful, loved, and at peace. It evokes all the emotions that you should always have right before bedtime, especially when your goal is to feel at ease.

Exercise

On this day, you'll move through a circuit of all five indoor exercises back-to-back with no rest in between.

- Start by performing the Double-Pump Shoulder Press for twelve repetitions.
- From there, you'll perform Dips for twelve repetitions.
- Next, you will do Squat & Holds for twelve repetitions.

- After that, you will do Step Ups for twelve repetitions (each leg).
- Finally, you'll get on the ground and do Bicycles for twenty repetitions.
- Rest for three minutes by walking (or standing) in place, then repeat the mini-circuit twice more for a total of three circuits.

Nutrition

Throughout Week Two, you made choices and changes in your life that served to elevate both your physical and spiritual bodies. One of the joys of the fasting process is the way it raises His voice, so that you may hear Him more clearly.

The noisiness of our lives can keep us bound to the things that hold us back. But as we fast, much of that commotion begins to fade away. We start to hear His voice more often and with greater clarity, and suddenly what He wants from us becomes more apparent.

You begin to hear His influence over your feelings of struggle, temptation, or whatever negative things are weighing on your mind. Consequently, elevating God's voice in our lives through fasting leads to an elevation in our faith and allows us to walk with more precision and certainty.

Also, by simplifying your diet to only a handful of things, you'll have more time to spend in thought, instead of always contemplating what your next meal may be. You're removing some of the distraction that can come from too many decisions to make, which will give you more time to listen to what He has to say.

DAY 39 (WEDNESDAY)

Concede

Father, I speak Your Word into my life. Show me its significance and how it has transformative power. Even when there is no Bible present, I want to know Your Word as if it was bound to my heart, so that no matter what, it will always be a part of me. Thank You, Father. Amen.

Honor

Finding the extra strength we may need to persevere can be as easy as going back to the Bible and really digging into its message. Joshua 1:8 is very specific about explaining the power of God's Word and how it can help us triumph over all obstacles:

> *"This Book of the Law shall not depart from your mouth, but you shall read it day and night, so that you may be careful to do in accordance with all that is written in it; for then you will make your way prosperous, and then you will be successful."*

Often we point our lives toward our earthbound desires. But as we turn to the Bible more often, the Word of God permeates us and guides us along more than any other earthbound desire. It becomes a part of our very essence, giving us a certain amount of strength and vitality that we cannot derive from anything else. We all need that reminder of how God's Word harnesses *real* power. When we continuously seek and find the spirit that's alive in His Word, it can inspire us, assure us—and change the trajectory of our lives.

Offer

On Day 35, I asked that you try to pray aloud because it gives your words more authority. That same principle applies to reading aloud to others, which is why I encourage you to give back today by reading to someone.

If you're not sure where to begin, start by contacting a local school, library, hospital, or church and ask if they are looking for volunteers to read to others. If that's not possible, reading to your children also counts, especially if you're not in the practice of doing so. If you don't have children of your own but have young children in your lives in the form of nieces, nephews, grandchildren, or children of close friends, offer to read them a bedtime story over Skype or FaceTime.

You don't have to read the Bible to someone else—and in some situations, that might not be allowed—but if you have that option, I encourage you to put some deep thought into which empowering scriptures you would like to share with them. Taking the time to read certain passages to others may not only allow them to understand God's messages a little better; it may also inspire a discussion of their meaning, which will only further connect them with the Word of God.

Sleep

Your electronic fast will continue this evening. I would like you to turn off all electronics a minimum of thirty to forty-five minutes before bedtime. During that time, just pick up your Bible and read whatever you wish. Let the spirit decide the page you turn to—and savor what it has to teach you.

Throughout Seven Sundays, I've presented certain scriptures that not only work well with the program, but verses that are close to my heart. And if you're not the type who turns to the Bible as often as you'd like, I hope that my sharing them has made you curious to explore your own Bible even further.

You see, every verse I've shared along this journey is a passage that I discovered along my walk with God. That's the thrill of reaching for the Bible and reading whichever pages you're compelled to turn to. Tonight you just may stumble upon a few verses that touch your spirit immediately or that stick with you for some reason yet to be explained.

If you wish, instead of turning to the Bible, you're also welcome to read through devotionals, Scripture-based periodicals or books, printed sermons, or anything that is truly in touch with what He has to say. The only condition I have is that whatever you read should be uplifting and peaceful, since the objective is not only to fill your spirit with the Word of God but to place you in a calm state of mind that's more prepared for sleep.

Exercise

Today is an Acknowledge-Pray-Rest Day. Allow your body to recover from what you accomplished on Days 37 and 38 by forgoing any form of strength-training exercise. However, if you wish to walk with God on this day, you may do so as long as your Worship Walk doesn't exceed thirty minutes and you maintain a relaxed, comfortable pace. If you wish to spend additional time with Him, I encourage you to spend that time in prayer to allow your body to recover and heal.

Nutrition

By following this strict intermittent fast, you're already embodying what Week Three was about (purification) through eating nothing but Faith-Full Foods. But from a spiritual standpoint, you're also purifying yourself of the power your flesh holds over your spirit. To help remind you of that fact, consider Matthew 26:40–41 on this day:

> *And He came to the disciples and found them sleeping, and said to Peter, "So, you men could not stay awake and keep watch with Me for one hour? Keep actively watching and praying that you may not come into temptation; the spirit is willing, but the body is weak."*

These two verses remind us that the spirit is always stronger than the flesh. As we fast, some of our significant temptations emerge to entice us. It's during this time that we are obviously lured to give in—and that's perhaps one of the greatest lessons gained through fasting.

It's about learning not to listen to that side of ourselves and instead heeding what the Spirit is telling us, which is to stay in this fast. It's telling us to stay true and remain connected to God.

What you're doing is breaking free from the enticements of the flesh so your spirit will grow stronger, but also so you can see that it is possible to overcome temptation through Him. Recognizing that you're no longer controlled by the flesh allows you to operate out of the fruits of the Spirit.

DAY 40 (THURSDAY)

Concede

Father, I yearn to have a relationship with You. I ask that You develop better relationship qualities within me so that I can build a stronger relationship with You, my family, and my friends. Guide my steps toward relationship and not religion. Set me free from transactional relationships and open me up to a deep connection with You. Thank You, Father. Amen.

Honor

If someone asked you to list everyone you know in the order of how much you love them, my guess is the list wouldn't be arranged in the order of how long you've known the person or how many moments you've spent with them. The order of your list wouldn't be based on numbers—it would be based on feelings. Someone you just met months ago could very well make the top of the list above others whom you've known your entire life.

The point is that what determines how close we are to someone isn't how much time we've put in with them—it's how far we've grown with them. That's what Acts 17:27 reminds us when it comes to becoming closer to God:

This was so that they would seek God, if perhaps they might grasp for Him and find Him, though He is not far from each one of us.

The difference between *religion* versus having a *relationship with God* is something that I've personally struggled with along my walk with Him—and it took me a while to understand that there's a difference.

I often have to release the bondage I have to the idea that if I do the right things, God will bless me. I have to remind myself that He isn't confined to this type of system, and instead understand how He looks at my heart and my love for Him. Because once I began to seek a relationship with God instead of strictly seeking to follow the rules I'd been taught about religion, my heart started to change, and all my relationships grew stronger as a result—especially my closeness to Him.

Religion shouldn't be all about "what you do" as a Christian—like following a routine and how well you can stick to it. Our God doesn't work that way, and how closely we walk with Him isn't based on any type of merit or performance. He has already told us that He loves us unconditionally, and he's waiting for us to find Him. All you need to do is let Him in.

Offer

God is always there for us when we need His guidance and support, so today think about offering that same guidance and support for someone by becoming a mentor.

If you believe you have nothing to offer, remember that you are further along than someone else. The wisdom we gain through age and experience is meant to be shared, and mentoring someone younger and less experienced doesn't have to be as imposing or impossible as it sounds. In fact, your obligation may only take minutes of your time.

It can be as easy as thinking about who in your life could use a little support to move forward, then letting them know you're always available for advice if they ever need it. Or if you can't find any opportunities on your own, try reaching out to any organization that pairs individuals with others who are in need of guidance, such as Big Brothers Big Sisters or the Mentoring Center (mentor.org).

I'm asking you to do this offering not just to give back to others—though that's a good goal—but because you'll receive from them as well. Sometimes we don't recognize our full value until we see how others welcome what we have to offer. Mentoring gives us that direct feedback—a sort of harvest, if you will—that validates and appreciates all the labor we've put in over the years, letting us see our true self-worth through the eyes of others.

Sleep

Tonight you'll turn off all electronics a minimum of forty to sixty minutes before bedtime. To fill that extra time, you can choose from all three things you've been doing over the last three evenings: praying longer, listening to Christian music, and reading the Bible.

God has blessed us with so many unique ways to grow closer to Him, so turn to whichever your spirit yearns for this evening. With all three options on the table, you'll reach for what's best for you to connect with Him. But if you would like, feel free to do all three—or even try them all at once.

Typically, when we bond with God in these traditional ways, we perform each of them separately. But often combining them can have a more significant impact on our spirit, and we may influence one another in unique and positive ways.

For example, you could listen to music as you pray or be inspired by the words you hear in a song to find and reread certain passages in the Bible. Or try reading the Bible with Christian music in the background, then stop between passages to share your thoughts on what you're reading with God through prayer. When you merge several different ways to connect with Him this evening, you may discover that you go further with Him spiritually than ever before.

Exercise

Today you'll Worship Walk for thirty minutes, then hike, bike, or swim—whichever activity you're most comfortable with—for twenty minutes (preferably outdoors, but using a stationary bike, treadmill, or indoor pool is fine if that's your only option).

If none of these options are possible, then you may perform a walk/jog workout instead of hiking, biking, or swimming. Start by walking at a leisurely pace for one to two minutes, then jog for thirty to forty-five seconds. Continue to alternate between walking and jogging for the duration of the workout (twenty minutes total).

Nutrition

Just as Week Four was all about adaptation, this week's fast is giving you yet another opportunity to adapt. Although performing this more stringent intermittent fast may feel like an unnatural process, it's one that forces us to eat as purely as possible by consuming only Faith-Full Foods.

Before Seven Sundays, your body was out of tune with the way God intended it to operate. But by eating only foods our bodies were meant to eat, we're returning our bodies to their original alignment. Think of how ironic that is—that your body is adapting to foods it was always meant to eat in the first place? Know that you'll come out the other side both spiritually stronger and physically healthier.

DAY 41 (FRIDAY)

Concede

Father, help me maintain my faith through the very end. I know You say that sustaining my belief will produce perseverance, but I feel like I'm hanging on by a thread and there's no evidence of progress. Show me that everything I'm doing is worth something; make my faith evident in my endurance and patience toward You. Thank You, Father. Amen.

Honor

With only a handful of days left, sustaining your faith can be the greatest hurdle of all. But as James 1:2–4 teaches us, what tests our faith should make us happy:

> *Consider it nothing but joy, my brothers and sisters, whenever you fall into various trials. Be assured that the testing of your faith produces endurance. And let endurance have its perfect result and do a thorough work, so that you may be perfect and completely developed, lacking in nothing.*

Know that everything you've done over the last forty days has fostered a faith in you that's stronger than before. Realize that the fruits of your labor will show soon enough if you haven't already seen them up until now. Maintain that faith and don't just persevere—but be elated.

These scriptures remind us to be joyful when we recognize that we are being tested. God strengthens our faith for a reason, so that we can be ready for whatever He has in store for us next. So, through your trials and tribulations, try to be jubilant and maintain that joy all the way until the end to prove to yourself what is possible.

Offer

This entire week—and all of Seven Sundays—calls upon you to rely on your faith to persevere. But perhaps no one relies on their faith more often than the brave men and women in the military.

Soldiers must have faith in their equipment, faith in the others serving around them, faith in their commanders, and faith that what they are doing is right and just. Most important of all, if they believe, they must have faith in God. That's why today I encourage you to send a care package to a soldier, to someone you most likely don't know nor will ever meet, but you are both bonded by one crucial thing—your faith. Just go to defense.gov/Resources/ and click on "Care packages" under the "Community" heading. From there, the US Department of Defense website will show you all the organizations you can contact, letting you know what's appropriate to send and exactly how to do so.

When soldiers get a random package from someone they may not know—some stranger who cared enough to put together something for them—it reminds them that people back home haven't forgotten them. You're showing someone that you appreciate what they're doing, what they're risking, and what they're sacrificing, all for your safety and freedom, as well as the safety and freedom of others.

You're also both building and maintaining faith in that one soldier. You may never know where their faith resided before receiving your package, but you can be confident that it will be bolstered when they open it.

Sleep

Your electronic fast will continue this evening as you turn off all electronics a minimum of sixty to seventy-five minutes before bedtime. You'll use that extra time to find out what God is saying to you—and through you—this evening. Sit down with nothing more than a few pieces of paper and something to write with, allow the Holy Spirit to come into you—and just write.

I could give you direction, or examples of what others have poured out onto the page close to the end of their journey, but that might influence the route you take. Instead just have faith that whatever you write is what needs to be written. No matter what you write, no matter how few words you scribble or how many pages you fill, trust that whatever pours out onto the page has found its way there for a reason. Just be in the moment with Him—and be excited to see what God reveals to you.

Exercise

On this day, you'll move through a circuit of all five indoor exercises back-to-back with no rest in between.

- Start by performing the Double-Pump Shoulder Press for twelve repetitions.
- From there, you'll perform Dips for twelve repetitions.

- Next, you will do Squat & Holds for twelve repetitions.
- After that, you will do Step Ups for twelve repetitions (each leg).
- Finally, you'll get on the ground and do Bicycles for twenty repetitions.
- Rest for one minute by walking (or standing) in place, then repeat the mini-circuit twice more for a total of three circuits.

Nutrition

Week Five was about glorifying Him, and what you're doing right now through fasting is extending that glorification. But as you do, keep in mind where that glory should be aimed. Matthew 6:17–18 reminds us:

"But when you fast, put oil on your head and wash your face so that your fasting will not be noticed by people, but by your Father who is in secret; and your Father who sees in secret will reward you."

Jesus reminds us that we should never fast for praise or to draw attention to ourselves. We're told to wash our face—meaning that we shouldn't be obvious about our fasting. This is all about glorifying God, not drawing attention to ourselves. But I also understand that it might be difficult this week in particular to deal with social situations. Just understand that if you have shared this part of your journey with others, that's okay.

As you take part in the Seven Sundays program, I'm confident that you're here with the right intentions. I feel confident that you've chosen this path not for the spotlight, but to spend more time alone with Him. So know this: Even if you've revealed to many people that you've been fasting, as long as you were sincere when discussing it (and never talked about it in a boastful or sorrowful way or to try to gain attention), it's understood. In fact, who knows—witnessing you glorifying God through fasting may eventually encourage others to do the same.

DAY 42 (SATURDAY)

Concede

Father, I surrender to You so that I may experience the fullness of life that stems from Your grace and mercy. Open my eyes to my enemy's ways so that I won't fall into his deceitful traps. Continue to shepherd me down the straight and narrow path to truth in life. Thank You, Father. Amen.

Honor

The inspiration for today's conceding comes from John 10:10, which is such an important verse to read on this final day before reaching your Seventh Sunday:

> *"The thief comes only in order to steal and kill and destroy. I came that they may have and enjoy life, and have it in abundance."*

You have gone through this journey for a fuller relationship with God, and over these past weeks, you've also become spiritually and physically stronger. You're at a different place where you can experience a fuller sense of life—and continue to do so—if you keep fostering that positive mentality.

But as far as we've come, we can just as easily fall backward if we let our recent successes cause us to become complacent. We all have the ability to slip back into a negative place within our minds and hearts. But when we remain aware that when those moments come, it's just the enemy trying to steal our joy and love, we can prevent that regression.

The Bible warns us of this thievery so that we may not only expect it but remember how to stop the theft and destruction. It tells us how we can always embrace the fullness of life by merely knowing the truth that only comes from knowing Jesus. He always walks along the path that leads to victory, so believe in Him always, and know that your walk with Him is both forever—and always pointing forward.

Offer

When we're able to connect people, we bring a sense of fullness not only to the two lives we have joined together but to our own. That's why the final offering of Seven Sundays is to share your relationships. It's about uniting two people you love and trust who don't know each other (or have never really had the chance to connect with each other) and who could benefit from being introduced.

Try playing matchmaker, but not necessarily from a love perspective. Think about it as networking for the spirit. It's about introducing two people who *should* know each other, who would *benefit* from knowing each other, and could have *fuller* lives by knowing each other.

Tomorrow you'll be reflecting upon how your relationship with God has grown and how that stronger relationship with Him has made your own life that much richer. You'll thoroughly grasp what comes from a stronger bond. And today you are the spark. You have the opportunity to make the world a little bit better by bringing together and improving the lives of two like-minded individuals.

Finally, if this task feels awkward, remember that you've chosen two people you're fond of and trust. Just explain how this task is part of your journey and that there's no pressure for anyone to break ground on a new friendship. It's the intention that matters most—the fact that you cared enough about both of them to try.

Sleep

On your final night of fasting from electronics, you will turn off all electronics a minimum of seventy-five to ninety minutes before bedtime—and spend all that time with your loved ones. Tonight don't just step away from electronics, but try asking those you're with to do the same.

When I say spend time with, I don't mean watching television together. This is about turning everything off—and *tuning in* to those around you. Spend this time doing anything you wish: having a conversation, playing a board game, sitting and watching the stars, listening to music, or just sitting together without speaking a word. Think of the things you never seem to have time for with them—and make that time.

If you live by yourself, then you're free to use technology to connect with someone, but try doing it in a personal way that also doesn't expose you to artificial light. That means no texting, e-mailing, or instant messaging, but using a phone for its primary function—to actually talk with someone.

If no one is awake or around tonight, then connect with those you love in other ways. That might mean breaking out a box of photographs of those you care about or looking at mementos and personal objects. It might mean cherishing past gifts, old cards, or anything that hasn't been appreciated in a while but connects you with someone you love. Whatever you choose, take this time to remind yourself how fortunate you are to know—and to have known—all the people in your life.

Before sleep, take a few seconds to recognize just how full and at ease your spirit should feel. What I love best about this night is how it proves to us how easy it is to carve out these heartfelt moments, day or night. All it takes is putting down what's in our hands and pulling in close those who are in our hearts.

Exercise

Today is an Acknowledge-Pray-Rest Day, and after such a hard week of exercise, enjoy this day because you've earned it. Allow your body to recover from what you accomplished on Days 40 and 41 by forgoing any form of strength-training exercise. However, if you wish to walk with God on this day, you may do so as long as your Worship Walk doesn't exceed thirty minutes and you maintain a relaxed, comfortable pace. If you wish to spend additional time with Him, I encourage you to spend that time in prayer to allow your body to recover and heal.

Nutrition

This is the last day of your modified intermittent fast, which in and of itself demonstrates your dedication to Him and exemplifies what this entire week has been about. To give you strength on this final day, remind yourself of the forty-day fast that Jesus undertook, as explained in Luke 4:1–2.

Now Jesus, full of the Holy Spirit, returned from the Jordan and was led by the Spirit in the wilderness for forty days, being tempted by the devil. And He ate nothing during those days, and when they ended, He was hungry.

As Christians, we are each called upon to become more like Jesus, and His fast was also a dedication to His Father. That said, I urge you not to think about today as one you hope will pass quickly, but a day that will last for as long as possible. For you are far from the end, but at the start of something new.

During your final morning of abstinence from food and through-out this evening when you stop eating until breakfast the next morning, relish these last few moments of your fast. Don't let these moments slip away—but savor them instead—for they are the final sacrifices you'll be making along the Seven Sundays journey. They are your last examples—for now—of your dedication to Him.

DAY 43 (SUNDAY)

THE SEVENTH SUNDAY

The Day of Completion
(Day 43)

On this final day, you'll reflect on your entire journey. But for now, begin the morning as you have every day throughout Seven Sundays—by surrendering to Him.

Concede

Father, I know that I'll never be a complete and perfect product, but I'm going to celebrate anyway because the victory resides in getting to know You more. I am going to let this newfound relationship with You give me confidence to take into the unknown. I'm going to allow all the fruits of the spirit to guide my life here forward. I now feel new in Christ. Thank You, Father, for everything You have done for me. Amen.

———

This walk with Him was never about the scale, being able to wear a smaller dress or pair of pants, or making your doctor pleased, even though I'm sure you're much happier with whatever numbers have changed along the way.

I understand that there may be physical changes that you're proud of, since losing unhealthy pounds is an inevitable (and enviable) effect of following Seven Sundays. And know that if you repeat the program, those changes will only continue for you (and I'll soon reveal how to embark on the next Seven Sundays). But for now, I want to focus on the main reason you took this journey, which was out of the desire for a deeper relationship with God. So tell me:

Where Are You Now—with Him?

Even if you were close to Him at the start, can you feel a difference? Is there more of a yearning in your heart for God?

For some of you, these questions may be easy to answer, but for others it may be hard to gauge. To help you recognize how far your relationship has grown, consider these questions:

- Do you feel more compelled to turn to the Word of God?
- Have you found yourself more eager to worship?
- Are you finding that you spend more minutes in the day praising Him than previously?
- Do you feel a sense of peace wash over you more often, particularly at times when you need it most?
- Do you find yourself more grateful and feel more content in your life?
- Did you end up repeating an offering you weren't asked to repeat—or looking back at certain concedings or honorings—simply because you wanted to?

Where Are You Now—with Others?

Now think about the people in your life.

- Is your relationship with each person the same as it was Seven Sundays ago, or even stronger now? Some relationships may remain the same, but I'm confident that others have improved as the result of your actions or because the people you know have watched you on your journey.
- Are there new people in your life who weren't there before? Somewhere along the way, I hope you've met someone new. What role that person will play in your life from this point forward is something only God knows. But what I know is that your new relationship began out of kindness and honesty—and that's not a bad place to start.

Where Are You Now—with Yourself?

This one I can answer for you: where you are now is where you're meant to be—for the moment, that is.

By taking this journey, your life is probably better. I don't have to know you personally to know that everything you've gone through has exposed you to many great opportunities to grow spiritually, physically, emotionally, and personally. You're a healthier person inside and out; you went through this for a reason, and now you're coming out the other side a better person. If you've faithfully followed the Seven Sundays program, I feel confident you'll have seen progress in your life:

- You'll have eliminated some of the distractions that have kept you from being as healthy as possible.
- You'll have begun the healing process on some of the wounds from your past.

- Do you feel more compelled to turn to the Word of God?
- You'll have initiated or recommitted to the act of prayer as part of your daily regimen and are now aware of new ways to make your talks with Him even more meaningful.
- You'll find yourself wanting to serve Him more and being more aware of when and where you're most needed.
- Your exercise and nutritional habits will have significantly improved, and as a result, you find yourself with more energy and ability.
- Your recovery habits have evolved in a way that not only helps your body heal but also helps your spirit grow. You're more relaxed before bedtime and more refreshed when waking up.
- You physically look more rejuvenated and relaxed.
- Your life will feel as if it is in better balance than before.
- You're a little less fearful and far more confident when stepping into a room or taking on a particular task or situation.
- You're more comfortable with your body—both physically and spiritually.

What If I Can't See What You See?

If some of these attributes aren't quite there yet, you'll get there. Even if you didn't achieve everything you wanted, reflect on what you were able to accomplish in a mere six weeks.

- Even if certain honorings held no meaning for you this time through, I hope others left an impression on your spirit.
- Even if you haven't managed to achieve every single offering, many lives have become much richer through the acts of kindness and generosity you did manage to complete.

- Even if your sleep habits aren't perfect, they're much improved, and because of that, so is your health, mind-set, appearance, and ability to heal.
- Even if you're not at your fittest or feeling entirely comfortable in your own skin, you've made changes both internally and externally. Some changes may not yet be revealed, while others could be changes you're not allowing yourself to see—for now.
- Even if you didn't manage to curb or eliminate every Faith-Less Food and incorporate every Faith-Full Food, you changed the ratio of healthy foods versus unhealthy foods in your diet in your favor.

Feeling like a failure for not reaching all your goals is a waste of effort, because you're already a success. You've made a difference over Seven Sundays, a difference that many Christians never reach within a year—or for some, within a lifetime. But even if something is preventing you from recognizing the difference you've made, that's understandable.

As Christians, we tend to embody humility because that's what we're called to do. I sometimes forget some of the ways that I've helped people throughout my journey share their feelings with me. But there is no hiding behind humility from what you've achieved over Seven Sundays—it's all there in black and white.

Go back and tally up every offering and see how many you were able to finish in so little time. Add up the number of people you met along the way, then ask yourself: If I hadn't taken this journey with Him . . .

. . . would those I had helped still be in need of help?

. . . would those I had shown kindness toward still be lost, sad, angry, or anxious?

. . . would those I had supported and encouraged still be in the same low place that I had lifted their spirits out of?

It's important to receive the praise for all the goodness you have done. Because even if just one person was motivated by watching you, even if just one person questioned their relationship with God simply by watching you along some point of your journey—wouldn't *that alone* have made the journey worth it?

God is always working behind the scenes, and although our work may not have been acknowledged, we should trust that what we've done has made a difference—and that we've planted a seed for the future. Each time you stepped outside to exercise with God, you may have motivated someone to start exercising for the first time that day. Any time you made a smarter choice with your nutrition, you may have made someone else rethink a Faith-Less Food and opt for a Faith-Full one instead. Even if you simply smiled at a stranger along the way, you may have brightened up someone's day just enough to change it.

After the Seventh Sunday . . .

My clients are often surprised when I explain how I continue to struggle and always need to remind myself of His blessings through prayer, fasting, and relying on the Pillars of Promise. But isn't that a pilgrimage that all true Christians take?

Seven Sundays is something you can repeat as many times as you like. The beauty of that is that each time you take the journey, you begin a little further along with Him than you were before. The more times you continue the program, the deeper your relationship with God will go—and the healthier your physical and spiritual bodies will become.

Before You Start Again . . .

Don't Rush Back in Too Fast. I really encourage you to let what you've learned over the last seven Sundays sink in. In fact, try spending a week allowing your life to take its normal course to see what happens. Many times, once a lifestyle program is over . . . well, it's over for most people. Without a game plan to follow, it's easy to slip back into your former habits, and you might do the same with certain ones that were more of a challenge for you. Allowing this time before you start again will help point out the areas where you struggle the most, so you can attack those areas with the greatest amount of authority the next time.

Think about Which Offerings Were the Most Difficult. There were some that probably took more preparation than you expected or more effort than you could manage at that moment. Take the time to skim through all the offerings and plan ahead if necessary, so that you can accomplish each offering precisely on the day you're meant to complete it.

Remember Your Weaknesses. If you're like most people, you've likely reduced your intake of Faith-Less Foods but didn't eliminate them altogether. Also, you most likely explored certain Faith-Full Foods, but either didn't incorporate them as often into your diet or didn't explore other options to try. When you do the program again, try to work on these areas even more.

Once You Start Again . . .

With the exception of a few slight modifications, simply start on the first Sunday (Day 1).

Concedings. The concedings in Seven Sundays came straight from my heart, but your relationship with God is unique—and so are the words you may want to share with Him at the start of each day. I encourage you to listen to what the Spirit is telling you: you can either say the concedings verbatim or use them as inspiration to come up with your own, from-the-heart way to surrender to Him.

Honorings. Because the Bible is meant to be read as often as possible, you're free to meditate on the same verses as well. In fact, what you'll find is that certain honorings may take on an entirely different meaning the more times you run through the program. If you like, make it a challenge to yourself each time to find additional pieces of scripture that match what you're going through that day. Other verses may help inspire you even more as you go along, and you may be in a different place spiritually and looking for something that speaks to you that day on a different level. In fact, I challenge you to do that each time you repeat the program because it will help you explore the Word of God in a way that's entirely different from simply reading the Bible on its own. But if that's too much work, sticking with each original honoring is fine as well.

Offerings. The beauty of Seven Sundays is that the offerings are evergreen. You can stick with the same ones for each day or challenge yourself to think of new offerings to try that you feel would have equal effect in growing your relationship with Him and making a difference in others' lives. If you stick with the same offerings, then I encourage you to remember how you tackled that offering the last time through, then try to figure out how you could make a more significant impact this time.

As for the Three Pillars that lead to a healthy physical body—sleep, exercise, and nutrition—you can still follow the program as is, especially when it comes to both sleep and nutrition.

Much of what you've learned along the way should still be a part of your routine. When you start Seven Sundays over again and come to the sleep and nutrition portions of each day, if you're already implementing what's being asked of you that day, give yourself a pat on the back for a job well done. And if you're not (or it's an area you're doing but could improve upon, such as cutting back even further on certain Faith-Less Foods), then look at each day as a reminder to do just that.

One question I'm always asked regarding this stricter version of intermittent fasting is how often it can be done. If you intend to repeat Seven Sundays immediately after completing the program, know that you can safely do so from a dietary standpoint. Because of the way the program is designed, you'll still be giving your body a monthlong break between each normal intermittent fasting and stricter intermittent fasting session.

As for the exercise portions, even though I don't know what your fitness level was before Seven Sundays, I am sure it's improved. Because of that, starting from the very beginning again may not be enough of a challenge, but know that you can modify the exercise portions accordingly:

- If the routine felt just right the last time through, then stick with the program as is.
- If there were specific exercises that required you to do the more forgiving version the last time through, then try to perform the exercise as described.
- If there were specific exercises that you did as described the last time through, then try to do the more aspiring version.

Finally, if the last time you explored Seven Sundays, you performed every exercise at their highest level (the aspiring versions), you have several options to try:

- You can stick with that program but perform each exercise at a slightly slower pace so that your muscles stay contracted for a longer period of time.

- You can repeat each circuit an additional time (for example, if you're asked to repeat the circuit for a total of three times, then try four).

- Or you're welcome to switch out any exercises you find less challenging for ones that work the same muscles but are more challenging for you.

No matter how you choose to try Seven Sundays your second, third—or even thirtieth time through—I can promise you this:

Your walk with Him will always be yours and yours alone. It is unlike any other walk others may take throughout Seven Sundays. Your journey will always be different from the last time, for even though you'll always be moving forward, the path you'll travel will always change. But I pray that one thing will always remain the same, no matter who you are or how many times you take this adventure with Him:

Your relationship with God will always be stronger at the end than when you began—no matter how close you were to Him when you started.

I'll see you next Sunday.

SEVEN SUNDAY EXERCISES

The ten exercises within the Seven Sundays program are each easily modified to match your current fitness level. When taking the journey, stick with the main exercise shown. However, if you find any exercise too difficult, you can try a variation of that exercise that's more *forgiving*. If you find any exercise too easy, you can try a variation of that exercise that's more *aspiring*.

OUTSIDE MOVEMENTS

Burpees

Prepare Yourself. Stand straight with your feet hip-width apart and your arms hanging straight down from your sides.

Perform the Movement. Quickly squat down and place your hands flat on the floor, then immediately shoot your legs straight behind you so that you end up in the top portion of a Push-up. Bend your elbows and do a quick Push-up; then without pausing, immediately jump your feet forward, so they land between your hands. Finally, stand back up. That's one repetition!

The Forgiving Option. You can make this easier in two ways: Instead of doing a traditional Push-up (with your legs straight), try resting on your knees instead. Another option: pause for a moment each time before continuing the exercise.

The Aspiring Option. Instead of just standing up at the end of each repetition to return to the start position, quickly jump up as high as you can with your arms extended above your head. As soon as you land, immediately squat down and repeat the exercise.

Lunges

Prepare Yourself. Stand straight with your feet hip-width apart. Raise your arms in front of you, make a fist with one hand, and cup your fist with the other, with elbows pointing out from your sides.

Perform the Movement. Take a big step backward with your left foot and lower yourself down by bending your right knee until your right thigh is parallel to the floor. Your left knee should almost graze the floor—but don't let it touch. Your goal should be to have both legs bent at a 90-degree angle. Push yourself back up into the starting position, then repeat, this time stepping back with your right leg. Continue to alternate from left to right for the duration of the exercise.

The Forgiving Option. Try a split lunge instead by standing in a staggered stance with your feet two and a half to three feet apart, left foot in front of your right. Lower your body until your left knee is bent 90 degrees; your right knee should nearly touch the floor. Push yourself back up into the starting position, then repeat. Once you've finished all the repetitions, repeat the exercise with your right foot in front of your left. Tip: If you can't lunge all the way down or have any problem balancing, place a chair alongside yourself and grab it for support as you perform the exercise.

The Aspiring Option. At the bottom of the movement, do a double pump by slowly raising up only a couple of inches, then sink back down into the lunge before pushing back up into the starting position.

Moving Planks

Prepare Yourself. Get yourself into a Push-up position with your arms straight, palms flat on the ground and spaced shoulder-width apart. Your legs should be extended straight behind you with your weight resting on your toes and the balls of your feet. Finally, pull in your stomach and tighten your core muscles.

Perform the Movement. Keeping your back straight, move your right hand to the left (placing your right hand next to your left hand) as you simultaneously step your left foot out to the left—your feet should now be wider than shoulder-width apart. Next, simultaneously move your left hand and right foot to the left so that you're back in the starting position.

Finally, reverse the exercise by traveling back to where you started. To do that, move your left hand to the right as you simultaneously step your right foot out to the right. Finish by simultaneously moving your right hand and left foot to the right so that you're back where you began.

The Forgiving Option. Instead of moving from side to side, you'll simply hold this position for the required amount of time. If that's too difficult, try bending your arms and rest on your forearms. Your elbows should be directly below your shoulders with your head facing down.

The Aspiring Option. After you've performed the moving plank twice (once to the left and to the right), try adding a Star

Plank in between. From the start position, twist your body to your right so that you're resting on the outside of your left foot. Reach your right arm up toward the sky and lift your waist away from the ground. You should be balancing on your left hand and the outside edge of your left foot. Finally, lift your right leg up as high as you can. Pause at the top, lower back down into the starting position, then repeat to the opposite side (this time by twisting your body to the left so that you're resting on the outside of your right foot, reaching your left arm up to the sky, then lifting your left leg up as high as you can).

Push-ups

Prepare Yourself. Get into position by placing your hands flat on the floor shoulder-width apart, then straighten your legs behind you with your weight on your toes. Your body should form a straight line from your head to your heels.

Perform the Movement. Keeping your head facing the floor, bend your elbows to lower yourself down, and stop once your upper arms are parallel to the ground. Immediately press yourself up by straightening your arms until you're back in the starting position.

The Forgiving Option. If you can't do a Push-up yet, try doing the movement with your knees on the ground. Or get into a Push-up position and lower yourself down to the ground as slowly as you can. It's fine if you can't push yourself back up. Instead do whatever's necessary to get yourself into a Push-up position, then repeat.

The Aspiring Option. Try to lower yourself down for a count of three to five seconds, then press yourself back up for a count of three to five seconds.

Supermans

Prepare Yourself. Lie flat on your stomach with your arms extended in front of you and your legs straight and together.

Perform the Movement. Keeping your head on the ground, slowly raise both arms and both legs at the same time. Hold the position at the top, then slowly lower your arms and legs back down into the starting position. That's one repetition!

The Forgiving Option. Instead of raising both arms and legs, slowly raise your left arm and right leg up at the same time. Hold at the top, slowly lower your arm and leg back down, then repeat—this time raising only your right arm and left leg up. That's one repetition!

The Aspiring Option. Keeping your head on the ground, slowly raise both arms and both legs up at the same time. Hold the position at the top, then slowly sweep your arms apart until they are extended straight out from your sides (from above, you should look like an airplane). Sweep your arms together in front of you once more, then slowly lower your arms and legs back down into the starting position. That's one repetition!

INSIDE MOVEMENTS

Bicycles

Prepare Yourself. Lie on the floor with your hands lightly cupped over your ears, elbows pointing out to the sides. Bend your legs and bring your knees up so that your thighs are perpendicular to the floor. Finally, lift your head and shoulders slightly off the floor.

Perform the Movement. Begin by slowly rotating your torso to the right, bringing your left elbow toward your right knee as you extend your left leg forward, keeping it elevated just off the floor. Reverse the motion by slowly rotating your torso to the left, bringing your right elbow toward your left knee as you extend your right leg forward (again, keeping it elevated just off the floor). That's one repetition. Continue to alternate from left to right, keeping your feet off the floor the entire time.

The Forgiving Option. If the cycling motion is too much for now, try knee raises instead. Lie flat with your arms down along your sides, knees bent, feet on the floor. Keeping your head, torso, and arms on the floor, slowly lift your pelvis up and curl your knees toward your chest as far as you comfortably can. Slowly reverse the motion to lower your feet back down to the floor. That's one repetition.

The Aspiring Option. Lie on the floor, then raise your arms and legs straight up so both your feet and hands point to the ceiling. Holding this position, slowly curl your torso up, twist to the left, and touch the outside of your right hand to the outside of your left ankle. Lower and repeat, this time twisting to the right and touching your left hand to your right ankle.

Dips

Prepare Yourself. Sit on the edge of a sturdy chair with your hands on the chair, palms down alongside your hips, knuckles facing forward. Position another chair directly across from you and place your feet on top. Shimmy your butt forward and off the seat until you're supporting your body's weight with your arms. Your knees should be bent with your heels down and toes up. This is the starting position.

Perform the Movement. Without moving your feet, slowly bend your elbows and lower your bottom down toward the floor until your arms are bent at a 90-degree angle. Your body should stay as close to the chair as possible as you go. Slowly press yourself back up until your arms are straight, elbows unlocked. That's one repetition!

The Forgiving Option. Instead of placing your feet up on a chair, just place them on the floor, keeping your legs either straight or with your knees slightly bent.

The Aspiring Option. If you have someone who can assist you, have them place either a light dumbbell or a weight plate on your lap directly over the front of your thighs. If you're exercising by yourself, try lowering yourself down for a count of three to five seconds, then pressing yourself back up for a count of three to five seconds.

Double-Pump Shoulder Presses

Prepare Yourself. Grab a dumbbell in each hand and stand in a staggered stance with your feet roughly eighteen inches apart, one foot forward and one foot back. (It doesn't matter which foot goes where—this position helps keep attention off the lower back—so take whatever stance feels natural.) Bend your arms and raise the weights up along the sides of your shoulders, palms facing forward, elbows pointing down.

Perform the Movement. Slowly squat down an inch or two, then stand up as you press the weights directly over your shoulders. At the top, don't let your elbows lock or bring the weights together at the top; they should move straight up instead. Slowly lower the weight back down to the sides of your shoulders. Finally, raise the dumbbells up an inch or two—this is the double pump—then lower them back down into the starting position. That's one repetition!

The Forgiving Option. Instead of standing in a staggered stance, stand straight with your feet hip-width apart and parallel to each other, weights held by your shoulders with your palms facing forward. Slowly press the weights straight up over your shoulders, but don't bring them together to touch at the top. Lower them back down to your shoulders—that's one repetition!

The Aspiring Option. Stand straight with your feet hip-width apart and parallel to each other with the weights held by your shoulders, palms facing into your body. Start the exercise by keeping the dumbbells by your shoulders as you slowly squat down until your thighs are almost parallel to the floor. Stand back up and press the weights directly over your shoulders. As you press, rotate the weights outward so that your palms face forward at the top of the movement. Lower the weights back down to the front of your shoulders, rotating them inward as you go so that you end up in the starting position. That's one repetition!

Squat & Holds

Prepare Yourself. Stand straight with your feet hip-width apart, toes pointed forward, and your arms hanging straight down at your sides, palms facing back.

Perform the Movement. Keeping your back flat, slowly squat down until your thighs are parallel to the floor, knees in line with your toes; don't let your knees move past your feet. As you squat, sweep your arms up in front of you and over your head so that your fingers are pointing to the ceiling at the bottom of the movement. Pause for three to five seconds, then press through your heels as you stand back up—and sweep your arms back down—into the starting position.

The Forgiving Option. Instead of squatting down all the way, try coming down only halfway to start, or try placing a chair behind yourself so you sit down and touch it after each repetition.

The Aspiring Option. There are a lot of different ways to make this move more difficult when you're ready. You can hold a dumbbell in each hand for added resistance, slow down how quickly you sink into the squat, pause at the bottom of the move for three to five seconds, or even do all three.

Step Ups

Prepare Yourself. Stand in front of a sturdy bench or chair with your feet shoulder-width apart, arms hanging down at your sides.

Perform the Movement. Keeping your back straight, place your left foot firmly on the bench and push yourself up (using only your left leg) until your right foot is able to step up on top of the bench—but don't place your right foot on the bench. Pause, then slowly lower your right foot back down to the ground so that it lands softly. Repeat for the required amount of reps, then do the exercise once more, this time by placing and keeping your right foot up on the bench.

The Forgiving Option. Instead of doing all the repetitions with one leg, then the other, do Alternating Step Ups instead by stepping up with your left leg first, then returning both feet to the floor, then stepping back up with your right foot. You can also try bringing both feet onto the bench after each step and pause for a second, which will give your muscles a quick rest in between.

The Aspiring Option. Perform the exercise holding a dumbbell in each hand for extra resistance.

ACKNOWLEDGMENTS

First and foremost, I want to thank God for this incredible journey that He has entrusted me with. If it wasn't for my relationship with Him, I would never have had the courage to step out of my comfort zone. God has revealed to me that there is much more in me than I could ever understand, and for that I am truly grateful. None of this would be possible without the abounding love and grace of God.

Second, I would like to thank Jay Schwartz not just for his friendship but also for his willingness to allow his own transformation to take place. Without your openness to allowing God to work through me, *Seven Sundays* might never have existed. You're an inspiration to me, and I look forward to embarking on this journey ahead with you.

Myatt Murphy: Thank you for being an awesome teammate on this project. You helped me push myself to higher levels and taught me not to be afraid of my own creativity. It's been a privilege to work with someone as creative and as talented as you. Thank you for your enthusiasm, diligence, and encouragement throughout this collaboration.

Heather Jackson: Thank you for taking a chance on this project, but most important, thank you for seeing the potential within me. I look back and connect the dots and realize that you have such a gift and a calling for what you do. It's been an honor to have you by my side; I feel unstoppable with such a loyal teammate fighting for me.

Beth Adams and the entire Howard team: Thank you for being so helpful and accommodating. This has been a wild ride with all of you. Words cannot express how excited I am to see God transform lives through *Seven Sundays*.

Eric (the Trainer) Fleishman: Thank you for giving me a shot when I first moved out to LA. I was innocent and naïve, but you saw something in me, and for that I'm honored to call you my friend and mentor. Everything I do and everything I become from here on out will bear your influence.

My family: Thank you for your love and prayers throughout this whole project. I couldn't have done it without you guys. I really believe that *Seven Sundays* will start a new path for our family and give birth to newfound hope for generations to come.

My friends (Natasha, Jonas, the Williams family, Carlos and Alexa, and Andrew): Thank you for pushing me to move forward with this book. When I didn't feel like I had anything left to give, you continued to support me. Your love was the foundation of my strength throughout this season of my life, and for that I am indebted.

NOTES

I: WHY IS CARING FOR YOURSELF SO HARD?

1. A. A. Shanb and E. F. Youssef, "The impact of adding weight-bearing exercise versus nonweight bearing programs to the medical treatment of elderly patients with osteoporosis," *Journal of Family & Community Medicine* 21, no. 3 (2014): 176–81, doi:10.4103/2230-8229.142972.

2. E. V. van Dongen et al., "Physical exercise performed four hours after learning improves memory retention and increases hippocampal similarity during retrieval," *Current Biology* 26, no. 13 (July 11, 2016): 1722–27, doi: 10.1016/j.cub.2016.04.071.

3. L. S. Pescatello et al., "American College of Sports Medicine position stand. Exercise and hypertension," *Medicine and Science in Sports and Exercise* 36, no. 3 (March 2004): 533–53.

4. Mayo Clinic, "Exercise helps ease arthritis pain and stiffness," https://www.mayoclinic.org/diseases-conditions/arthritis/in-depth/arthritis/art-20047971.

5. American Diabetes Association, "Fitness," http://www.diabetes.org/food-and-fitness/fitness/.

6. National Cancer Institute, "Physical activity and cancer," https://www.cancer.gov/about-cancer/causes-prevention/risk/obesity/physical-activity-fact-sheet.

7. Mayuree Rao et al., "Do healthier foods and diet patterns cost more than less healthy options? A systematic review and meta-analysis," *BMJ Open* 3, no. 12 (December 5, 2013): e004277, doi: 10.1136/bmjopen-2013-004277.

8. US Department of Agriculture, "USDA and EPA join with private sector, charitable organizations to set nation's first food waste reduction goals," Release no. 0257.15, https://www.usda.gov/media/press-releases/2015/09/16/usda-and-epa-join private-sector-charitable-organizations-set.

3: THE PILLARS OF PROMISE

1. Luciana Besedovsky et al., "Nocturnal sleep uniformly reduces numbers of different T-cell subsets in the blood of healthy men," *American Journal of Physiology* 311, no. 4 (2016): R637.

DAY 2

1. Diane S. Lauderdale et al., "Sleep duration: How well do self-reports reflect objective measures? The CARDIA Sleep Study," *Epidemiology* 19, no. 6 (November 2008): 838–45.

DAY 3

1. National Sleep Foundation, "Americans' bedrooms are key to better sleep according to new National Sleep Foundation poll," January 25, 2011, https://sleepfoundation.org/media-center/press-release/americans-bedrooms-are-key-better-sleep-according-new-poll.

DAY 6

1. M. Shin et al., "The effects of fabric for sleepwear and bedding on sleep at ambient temperatures of 17°C and 22°C," *Nature and Science of Sleep* 8 (April 22, 2016): 121–31.

DAY 9

1. V. Morhenn et al., "Massage increases oxytocin and reduces adrenocorticotropin hormone in humans," *Alternative Therapies in Health and Medicine* 18, no. 6 (November–December 2012): 11–18.
2. American Heart Association, "Whole grains and fiber," http://www.heart.org/HEARTORG/HealthyLiving/HealthyEating/HealthyDietGoals/Whole-Grains-and-Fiber_UCM_303249_Article.jsp#.Wgi1HLaZN0I.

DAY 10

1. A. T. Erkkila and A. H. Lichtenstein, "Fiber and cardiovascular disease risk: How strong is the evidence?" *Journal of Cardiovascular Nursing* 21, no. 1 (January–February 2006): 3–8.

2. J. M. Gutierres et al., "Neuroprotective effect of anthocyanins on acetyl-cholinesterase activity and attenuation of scopolamine-induced amnesia in rats," *International Journal of Developmental Neuroscience* 33 (April 2014): 88–97, doi: 10.1016/j.ijdevneu.2013.12.006, Epub December 24, 2013.

3. A. Karlsen et al., "Anthocyanins inhibit nuclear factor-kappaB activation in monocytes and reduce plasma concentrations of pro-inflammatory mediators in healthy adults," *Journal of Nutrition* 137, no. 8 (August 2007): 1951–54.

4. A. Gajowik and M. M. Dobrzynska, "Lycopene—antioxidant with radio-protective and anticancer properties: A review," *Roczniki Panstwowego Zakladu Higieny* 65, no. 4 (2014): 263–71.

5. O. Benavente-Garcia and J. Castillo, "Update on uses and properties of citrus flavonoids: New findings in anticancer, cardiovascular, and anti-inflammatory activity," *Journal of Agricultural and Food Chemistry* 56, no. 15 (August 13, 2008): 6185–205.

6. G. Ruel et al., "Favourable impact of low-calorie cranberry juice consumption on plasma HDL-cholesterol concentrations in men," *British Journal of Nutrition* 96, no. 2 (August 2006): 357–64.

DAY 12

1. K. J. Royston and T. O. Tollefsbol, "The epigenetic impact of cruciferous vegetables on cancer prevention," *Current Pharmacology Reports* 1, no. 1 (February 1, 2015): 46–51.

2. Rose K. Davidson et al., "Sulforaphane represses matrix-degrading proteases and protects cartilage from destruction in vitro and in vivo," *Arthritis & Rheumatology* 65, no. 12 (December 2013): 3130–140, doi: 10.1002/art.38133.

3. O. Sommerburg et al., "Fruits and vegetables that are sources for lutein and zeaxanthin: The macular pigment in human eyes," *British Journal of Ophthalmology* 82, no. 8 (August 1998): 907–10.

4. American Optometric Association, "Lutein & zeaxanthin," http://www.aoa.org/patients-and-public/caring-for-your-vision/diet-and-nutrition/lutein?sso=y.

DAY 14

1. E. J. Sung and Y. Tochihara, "Effects of bathing and hot footbath on sleep in winter," *Journal of Physiological Anthropology and Applied Human Science* 19, no. 1 (January 2000): 21–27.

2. National Institutes of Health: National Center for Complementary and Integrative Health, "Garlic," https://nccih.nih.gov/health/garlic/ataglance .htm.

3. British Psychological Society, "Rosemary aroma may help you remember to do things," *ScienceDaily*, April 9, 2013.

4. T. Allahghadri et al., "Antimicrobial property, antioxidant capacity, and cytotoxicity of essential oil from cumin produced in Iran," *Journal of Food Science* 75, no. 2 (March 2010): H54–61. K. S. Muthamma Milan et al., "Enhancement of digestive enzymatic activity by cumin (*Cuminum cyminum L.*) and role of spent cumin as a bionutrient," *Food Chemistry* 100, no. 3 (October 1, 2008): 678–83. K. Patel and K. Srinivasan, "Digestive stimulant action of spices: A myth or reality?" *Indian Journal of Medical Research* (May 2004).

5. Isabella Savini et al. "*Origanum vulgare* induces apoptosis in human colon cancer caco$_2$ cells," *Nutrition and Cancer* 61, no. 3 (2009): 381–89. Bonn University, "Salutary pizza spice: Oregano helps against inflammations," *ScienceDaily*, June 26, 2008.

6. B. Qin et al., "Cinnamon: Potential role in the prevention of insulin resistance, metabolic syndrome, and type 2 diabetes," *Journal of Diabetes Science and Technology* 4, no. 3 (May 2010): 685–93.

DAY 16

1. A. Jaehne et al., "Effects of nicotine on sleep during consumption, withdrawal and replacement therapy," *Sleep Medicine Reviews* 13, no. 5 (October 2009): 363–77.

DAY 18

1. O. I. Emilsson et al., "Respiratory symptoms, sleep-disordered breathing and biomarkers in nocturnal gastroesophageal reflux," *Respiratory Research* 17, no. 1 (September 20, 2016): 115.

2. Y. I. Fujiwara et al., "Association between dinner-to-bed time and gastroesophageal reflux disease," *American Journal of Gastroenterology* 100, no. 12 (December 2005): 2633–36.

3. World Health Organization, "WHO calls on countries to reduce sugars intake among adults and children," http://www.who.int/mediacentre /news/releases/2015/sugar-guideline/en/.

4. American Health Association, "Frequently asked questions about sugar," http://www.heart.org/HEARTORG/GettingHealthy/NutritionCenter

/HealthyEating/Frequently-Asked-Questions-About-Sugar_UCM
_306725_Article.jsp.

DAY 19

1. A. G. Harvey and S. Payne, "The management of unwanted pre-sleep thoughts in insomnia: Distraction with imagery versus general distraction," *Behaviour Research and Therapy* 40, no. 3 (March 2002): 267–77.

DAY 29

1. Min Wei et al., "Fasting-mimicking diet and markers/risk factors for aging, diabetes, cancer, and cardiovascular disease," *Science Translational Medicine* 9, no. 377 (February 15, 2017): eaai8700.